Pathways into caring

Judith Irving
Susan Munday
Ashley Rowlands

Stanley Thornes (Publishers) Ltd

First published in 1993 by:
Stanley Thornes (Publishers) Ltd
Ellenborough House
Wellington Street
Cheltenham
GL50 1YD
UK

A catalogue record for this book is available from the British Library.
ISBN 0 7487 1569 X

Typeset by Quorum Technical Services Ltd, Cheltenham
Printed and bound in Great Britain by Scotprint Ltd, Musselburgh

Acknowledgements

The authors and publishers are grateful to the following for permission to reproduce material in this book:

page 2, The Hutchison Library/Nancy Durrell McKenna; pages 7 and 14, Sally and Richard Greenhill; page 21, Photofusion/Vicky White; pages 37 and 46, Sally and Richard Greenhill; page 47, Network/Denis Doran; page 67, Aquarius Picture Library; page 73, Hulton-Deutsch Collection; page 76, Sally and Richard Greenhill; pages 9, 79, 81, 82, 83 and 84, HMSO © Crown; page 94, Sally and Richard Greenhill; page 105, Age Concern/J. Birdsall; page 107, Photofusion/Vicky White; page 116, The Hutchison Library/ Michael Macintyre; page 119, Tony Stone Worldwide/Loren Santow; page 135, Photofusion/Janis Austin; pages 143, 161, 164 and 185, Sally and Richard Greenhill. The charts from *Social Trends* are reproduced with the permission of the Central Statistical Office and are © Crown.

Every effort has been made to contact copyright holders, and we apologise if any have been overlooked.

Contents

Introduction

The 1980s has seen unprecedented change in what is known as the care sector, that is those areas of work associated with those who have some special need, be it poor health, learning difficulty or some other disability or dependency. This change has largely been brought about by government legislation which itself reflects a changing approach to the welfare of the population. In particular there has been a drift away from statutory welfare provision, as defined in the welfare legislation of the late 1940s, to more voluntary and private care. A parallel development has been the move towards more community-based care and greater emphasis on the rights of the service user – the patient, the elderly person in a residential home etc. – to define what service they want.

These developments will be referred to later in this book; however, the book's main purpose is to provide a practical, skills-related introduction to the knowledge base that any professional caregiver will need to operate effectively in their chosen job. Unfortunately the care sector has typically not given much attention to the training needs of staff who are not professionally qualified, nurses or social workers for instance. In fact, 80 per cent of all staff working in care have no formal training or qualification in this particular field. This situation is starting to change, however, with the arrival of National Vocational Qualifications (NVQs). The NVQs are a framework of qualifications cutting across all vocational sectors, which are based not on the acquiring of knowledge in an academic setting, but on the performance of job competence in the workplace using nationally agreed standards. They present exciting opportunities for employers and employees to extend the range of training, and the number of people benefiting.

This book has been written with one eye on the progress of NVQs. However, at the time of writing the situation is unclear as to exactly how the NVQs will affect the development of training, especially the area we shall refer to as pre-service. The pre-service group comprises all those individuals, whether school leavers or adults, who wish to do caring work below the level of the fully qualified professional. It is unlikely that this group will have direct access to the NVQs until they are in work, because of the difficulty in providing adequate work experience to enable the testing of competent performance to take place. To bridge the gap between the NVQ and the purely academic, subject-based approach the government is supporting the development of a General National Vocational Qualification (GNVQ) in each vocational area. This will have similar levels to the NVQ and will become the blueprint for the broad preparatory programmes such as the BTEC First and National awards, and the City and Guilds certificates. The GNVQ units will correspond approximately to the NVQs, but will only relate to the underpinning knowledge detailed in the NVQs. As a result of these developments this book has concentrated on covering the units currently prescribed by the Health and Social Care GNVQs.

It is necessary, therefore, for clarification as to the purposes of this book. First, it is expected that its readers will be following either a pre-service course leading to a recognised care certificate, or diploma or possibly an NVQ training programme. There is a difference between the person who needs a general introduction to the issues of care practice, and the more task-specific text which can be directly related to a particular client group and care setting. The task for the authors has been to provide a text which can meet the needs of both. Finally, this book does not have any direct reference to child care; in the NVQ structure there are separate standards for child care which will require different treatment and another book.

As the preceding comments will have indicated, this book is intended to provide a knowledge base, while at the same time encouraging the reader to explore the applications of the information provided and to read further to broaden their knowledge. In an introductory text such as this it is difficult to give a lot of detail in some, if not all, of the various topics. To help the reader's understanding and to broaden their knowledge of the topics you will find a number of different aids:

- *Case studies* – these are short accounts of real events or situations intended to illustrate the points being made in the main body of the chapter at that time.
- *To dos* – these are exercises designed to encourage further research into a subject, as well as providing a stimulus for discussion in the classroom situation. References are also made to other books or articles which may be of help in background reading.
- *Key points* – at the end of each chapter a summary of the key points is provided and at the end of the book a glossary of terms is included to help the reader chart their way through the mysterious waters of NHS and social services jargon.

At the time of writing there a number of good texts which provide an introduction to care settings or care practice. These tend to be geared towards the 'hands on' needs of people who are already in work, as care assistants, for instance. There are also many general texts which look at sociological, health or human development issues from a more academic perspective, perhaps preparing the reader for a GCSE or A level in that subject. This book is different in that it bridges the divide between the two approaches, and sets the information provided in a practical or work-based context.

We start with an introduction to the caring task by asking who the various service user groups who have special needs are. Reference is also made to the different settings in which these groups are found. The theme of the second and third chapters is the nature of the service provided to those in need. The services available are described by separating those that are institutionally based from those operating within the community. In each case attention is given to the differences between statutory, voluntary and private forms of care. In Chapter 4 the book shifts to explore some of the wider human and social issues concerning the service user. It is important for the caregiver to be aware of the background to the social problems that they encounter. This chapter outlines the role of the family, and of the socialisation process in general, in determining life chances. Following on from this, Chapter 5 outlines the role of the state in creating (or failing to create) a safety net for those who become dependent. It charts the progress of welfare from the Victorian era, when 'Let heaven help those who help themselves' was the dominant attitude, to the welfare state of the 1950s onwards.

The second half of the book devotes itself more to the practical skills involved in caregiving. Chapters 6 and 7 look at communication skills – written and oral – and interpersonal skills, respectively. The last three chapters concentrate on the physical and psychological needs of the individual, and some of the skills needed in assessing and meeting these needs.

In summary, then, this book will provide the reader with a broad and comprehensive introduction to the skills and knowledge base needed to become a successful caregiver. In many areas the book cannot go into sufficient detail to provide the necessary underpinning knowledge for some more specific vocational areas. The diversity of the caring situation – service user and care settings – will require the reader to extend their understanding through further reading. Nevertheless, this book offers an important start on the road to competence and qualification.

GNVQ level 2: Health and social care units

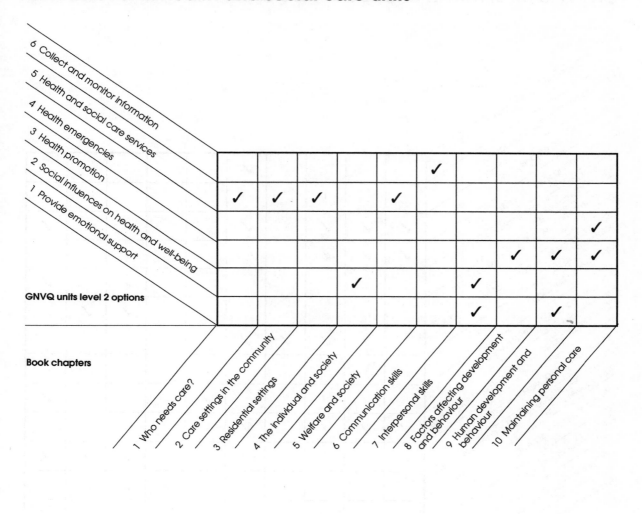

GNVQ units level 2 options / Book chapters	1 Who needs care?	2 Care settings in the community	3 Residential settings	4 The individual and society	5 Welfare and society	6 Communication skills	7 Interpersonal skills	8 Factors affecting development and behaviour	9 Human development and behaviour	10 Maintaining personal care
6 Collect and monitor information						✓				
5 Health and social care services	✓	✓	✓		✓					
4 Health emergencies										✓
3 Health promotion								✓	✓	✓
2 Social influences on health and well-being				✓			✓			
1 Provide emotional support							✓		✓	

GNVQ level 3: Health and social care units

GNVQ units level 3+ options	1 Who needs care?	2 Care settings in the community	3 Residential settings	4 The individual and society	5 Welfare and society	6 Communication skills	7 Interpersonal skills	8 Factors affecting development and behaviour	9 Human development and behaviour	10 Maintaining personal care
15 Understanding the development of social policy					✓					
14 Environmental safety and security										✓
13 Working in care organisations	✓	✓	✓		✓					✓
12 Understanding special needs	✓	✓	✓					✓		
11 Physiological and inheritable aspects of health and well-being								✓		✓
10 Human behaviour in the context of health and social care								✓	✓	
9 Social change in the context of health and social care		✓	✓	✓	✓					
8 Information handling						✓				
7 Health and social care delivery plans		✓				✓				✓
6 Structure and practices in health and social care	✓	✓	✓		✓					
5 Health and social well-being promotion								✓	✓	✓
4 Interaction between social, psychological and physical well-being				✓			✓	✓	✓	
3 Physical aspects of health								✓		✓
2 Interpersonal interaction							✓			✓
1 Access to health and social care				✓			✓			

Book chapters

1 *Who needs care?*

Everyone within our communities needs to be cared for in one way or another. This chapter is going to look at people within communities and the type of care they need at different stages of their lives. Some people will need high levels of care for all of their lives, e.g. people with chronic illness or disability, while others will need high levels at different points, with low levels of demand for the rest of their lives.

Who does the caring is another aspect that will be mentioned in this chapter, but detailed descriptions of organisations and the carers will be found in the next two chapters. It should be stated here that most caring is provided within the family by informal carers. At the beginning of the 1990s it was estimated that 6 million people, that is over 14 per cent of the population of the UK, received informal care in their home. Informal care refers to the care that is given by members of the immediate family, other relatives or friends. They may not have received any care training and are not usually professionally qualified. The care services either support that family care or they may replace it when a family can no longer be the main provider or it does not possess the necessary skills.

Care can mean many different things and there are many ways in which it can be given. It may mean providing support, supervision, training, physical or psychological care, counselling, or protection and safety.

The care providers

Care can be provided by many individuals and organisations in a variety of different settings. Care organisations can be defined as:

- statutory;
- voluntary; or
- private.

Statutory

Different government departments are responsible for statutory organisations (see charts outlining these structures in the appendix), the structures of which are laid down by law. They are designed to protect vulnerable groups of people and to provide services for them. For example, social service departments provide statutory services.

Voluntary

Statutory organisations are assisted in their tasks by a variety of voluntary organisations. They are not set up by law, but because individual founders see a need for a particular service, which often means that voluntary schemes

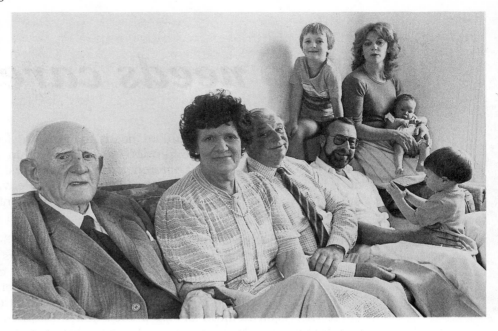

Most caring is provided within the family by informal carers.

are tailor-made for the needs of a particular group of people. They can be organised in several different ways.

● *Local* A group set up by local people, for example a youth club.
● *National* Usually having a central office, and local branches throughout the country. The following are two examples:

The **Samaritans** are an organisation providing a listening helpline to people who are desperate and feel they have no one to turn to.

Citizen's Advice Bureaux provide advice centres across the UK, offering specialist help in a variety of areas such as legal and financial. CABX also direct people to other organisations that can provide advice, support or care.

Voluntary organisations are run on a non-profit-making basis, and although they may receive help from volunteers, they may also employ people to provide the service.

Private

The UK also has a variety of private or profit-making organisations that provide care. In such cases, someone has again identified a need, but makes a business from fulfilling this need. There does, of course, have to be a market for these services, which means that they are only provided in areas for which people are willing to pay for the service. Private hospitals, residential homes and schools are examples, where people are willing to pay for what they often see as a better service than that which is provided by the statutory sector.

Community care plans

This diverse network of service providers has often led to problems in provision, which can mean that service users do not always enjoy the full benefits of the services provided in their locality. To try and overcome some of these problems, the government in 1990 introduced the National Health Services and Community Care Act, which provides a framework in which all the care providers, statutory, voluntary and private, can work together in a 'mixed economy of care'. This has meant that social service departments have had to co-ordinate and draw up community care plans for their areas, detailing how care is going to be provided for all the different user groups, and who is involved in providing that care. Local authorities will implement these plans from April 1993 onwards.

The subject of child care up to the age of seven years is a large one and will not be discussed in this book. The following user groups will be employed when discussing those receiving care:

- children over seven years;
- young adults;
- adults;
- elderly people;
- people with health problems;
- people with disabilities.

To do

Make a note of the different aspects of care you and your family have received. Write down who were the carers providing the care. Examples may include school, youth clubs, hospital care. Keep your notes for a later exercise.

Children seven years+

All children in the UK are entitled to receive, as their right, many different aspects of care including education and health care. The main points of change or stress experienced by a child after the age of seven are:

- changing school, usually between the ages of 11 and 13;
- the onset of puberty;
- peer group pressure.

For some there may be other stresses caused by conflict within the family, bereavement, accidents or socially-related problems such as smoking and substance abuse.

The services provided for children will now be discussed below.

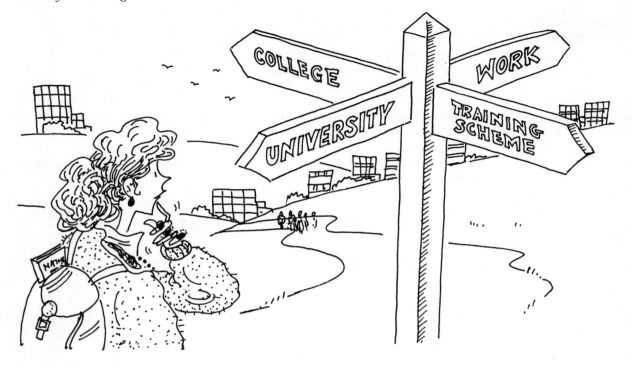

Education

In the UK it is compulsory for *all* children between the ages of 5 and 16 years to receive education, with every child being entitled to receive this as a free service. Some parents decide to opt out of the free provision and elect to pay for their children to attend private rather than state schools, or they may decide to educate their children at home.

Once the child has reached the age of 16, education is no longer compulsory, but is still provided as a free service, either at schools or at colleges, until the child reaches 19 years. Education and training is provided after this age, but is not a free right for everyone. People may attend colleges or universities at any stage of their lives, sometimes receiving some financial help, but others paying their own way. Alternatives to full-time education include training schemes where the individual receives a training allowance and, by working with an employer, receives training for a particular job. These schemes usually involve some theoretical as well as practical training, and there is usually an opportunity to obtain a qualification.

Health

Different health authorities throughout the UK will provide some preventative measures through school health services in order to protect children from illness or to help in the early detection of conditions that may require specialist help. Examples of these are the immunisation or vaccination programmes, and the medical and dental examinations that are carried out free of charge.

To do

Collect data from within your group about the vaccinations or immunisations you have received and construct a bar chart to illustrate your findings. Discuss the purpose of the vaccinations. Did you all receive a similar programme? If not, what are the reasons for the differences?

Social services

Social services aim to provide support services for those children with needs that cannot be met within their immediate families. For orphans or children whose parents, for one reason or another, are unable to care for them, social services can provide care, either in adoptive or foster homes, or within a residential care setting. Social service personnel also provide protection for young people who live at home, but who may be at risk. They can also act as advisers for young people with worries or anxieties, or for their parents.

Other

Several voluntary or charitable groups, such as the NSPCC or the National Children's Bureau, are also involved in some aspects of child care. These may offer protection, help or advice. In recent years there has been a greater awareness of child abuse, and Childline, a national telephone helpline, has been set up to help those children who do not know where or how to get help.

Other organisations offer services for all children who want to take part on a voluntary basis. These provide care in the sense of offering children opportunities to develop skills they might not gain within their families. Sports clubs run by volunteers, and organisations such as the girl guide and boy scout movements are examples of these.

Young adults

For the purposes of this chapter young adults are people who have reached the age of 18 and/or have left home. The main points of change for them are:

- leaving school at 16, 17 or 18 years;
- starting higher education or professional training;
- starting work.

As previously mentioned they may still be receiving some education services, although they (or their parents) may now have to pay for them.

Health

Young people can obtain advice on health issues from such places as health centres, health education departments and chemists. This advice can be on

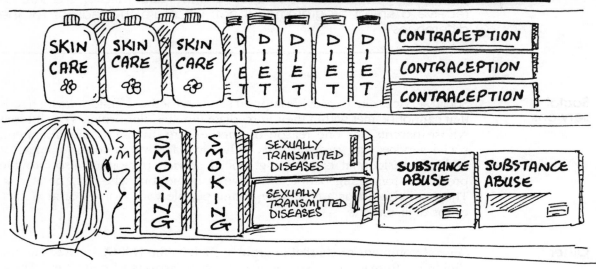

such matters as skin problems, diet, contraception (family planning), substance misuse, smoking or sexually transmitted diseases.

Social services

People who work for social services can provide advice and help with many problems that may occur, including housing problems and help with application for benefits.

Probation service

Young people who break the law and are convicted of an offence may come under the care of the probation department. Young offenders may receive a sentence which involves them remaining in the community, under the supervision of the probation service. One of the main aims of the probation service is to help offenders to remain in the community and not to reoffend.

Others

There are many other organisations involved with this group, some voluntary and some statutory, that can help with a whole range of problems, either of individuals or their relationships. Again, some voluntary groups help to provide facilities like youth clubs where young people can meet together in a safe environment.

To do

Either as an individual or in a group, list all the agencies that you can think of that are involved with young adults, and what they offer. Keep for reference in your future work.

Adults

During adult life there are many potential points of change. People will be affected differently, with some experiencing few changes, others experiencing many. Some of the changes that may occur are:

- changing jobs;
- promotion at work;
- being made redundant or retiring;
- relationships;
- marrying;
- having a family;
- divorce;
- bereavement;
- addiction problems.

Some of these events can create changes in lifestyle, such as poverty, which itself may cause other problems like homelessness. The range of service requirements for this category of clients is very wide.

Health

There are many times during an adult's life when they may need to call on the health services, either for advice or for help. The most obvious time is when they are ill, and these services will be detailed later. Increasingly, though, adults are now getting involved with preventive care, such as that provided at well-man or woman clinics, ante and post-natal clinics for mothers before and after the birth of their babies, and stress clinics.

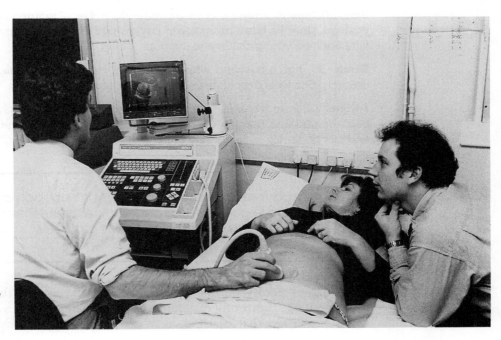

Ultrasound scans are now a routine feature of ante-natal care.

Social services

Social workers are available for advice on a variety of issues, and they may also give help at times of crisis, such as homelessness, when they can find accommodation for families.

Probation service

When adults are convicted of a crime they may receive a sentence which enables them to remain in the community. For more serious offences, or for those who repeatedly offend, a custodial or prison sentence may be passed. Those offenders remaining in the community, or those released from prison, are supervised and cared for by officers from the probation service.

Housing departments

These are part of district councils and are responsible for providing some housing for certain groups, including some homeless people, especially families.

Others

There are many agencies available to help with a variety of problems that can occur during adult life. These may be health or social problems, and relationship or family problems. For example, Relate is a voluntary organisation that is increasingly involved with a whole range of relationship problems, not just between married people. Other important advice and help centres are Citizen's Advice Bureaux and the Samaritans.

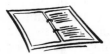

─────────── **Case study** ───────────

A community contains the following individuals, each with a different problem.

Mary, 46, has been feeling unwell for some months now. She is frequently tired, has headaches and is finding it difficult to hold down her job.

Ben, 26, has recently been made redundant. He is worried about his financial position, since he has a mortgage to pay, as well as hire-purchase payments, and a wife and two young children to support.

Sarah, 36, has a husband who is alcoholic. He has been violent to her and the children. She feels desperate and alone with no one to help her.

Fatima, 22, a student, has been evicted by her landlord, although she had regularly paid the rent and met the terms of her tenancy agreement. She is now homeless and has no family in the locality of the university.

To do

To which organisations would you suggest that each of the individuals described above goes for help and advice about their problem? Why? What help can these different agencies provide?

Elderly people

The phrase 'elderly people' normally refers to people who have reached retirement age, currently 60 years for women and 65 years for men. It must be remembered that many elderly people are fit, healthy and very able,

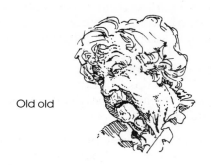

Old old

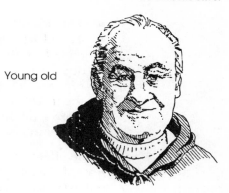

Young old

requiring little special help. With many people now living well into their 80s or even 90s this user group is now divided into the 'young old' and the 'old old'. The young old are people aged 60 to 75 years and the old old are people over 75 years. The old old are often referred to as the vulnerable old in that they are especially at risk from physical, psychological and social traumas.

The following table illustrates the trends in the elderly population, with information gathered from the 1981 census from the Office of Population Censuses and Surveys.

Trends in the ageing population

Census date			(projections)	
	1961	1981	1991	2001
Number by age (millions)				
65–74	3.9	5.0	5.0	4.6
75–84	1.8	2.6	3.0	3.0
85 and over	0.3	0.6	0.8	1.0

Just because a person has reached a certain age does not mean that they always become totally dependent on others. Individuals from any of these categories may be fit and able, making very few demands on the service providers. However, many people do develop either health or social problems as a result of the ageing process or a change in their life pattern, such as retirement.

The ageing process may affect many different parts of the body, either singly or they may have a cumulative effect, with one deficiency causing another. For example, pain from arthritis may prevent a person from consuming a balanced diet, because of the problems with shopping and cooking.

Some effects cannot be prevented but others can be delayed if not prevented altogether. There are many factors that influence the ageing process and the effects on different people. These include:

- *genetics* – the tendencies inherited from our parents;
- *wear and tear* – the wearing out of body tissues;
- *lifestyles* – the habits people adopt during their lives and the work they do;
- *illness* – developing at any stage of life;
- *social factors* – stress, relationships, culture;
- *work* – different occupations may be more likely to increase wear and tear, and also cause some illnesses.

Some effects, such as the hair turning grey or white, or men going bald, do not physically affect people's lives, although some people may react emotionally to these outward signs of ageing.

To do

Consider the changing pattern of the elderly population. What factors do you think are responsible for this? Suggest the implications for the service providers and how these could be incorporated into community plans.

The ageing process and the conditions arising from it are dealt with in detail in Chapter 9. Elderly people will have use of many services that have already been described, but they may have more specialised demands than those of other groups.

Health

This service will include the supply of any drugs that may be necessary to alleviate any of the symptoms caused by conditions such as arthritis. It also includes treatments such as physiotherapy and occupational therapy to help overcome some of the physical problems. It may provide hospital care for those people who need high levels of treatment or care, either in the short term or for longer periods.

Dental and chiropody services are also provided, together with help for those whose sight and hearing may have become impaired.

There is also provision for those who need occasional specialist help in their own homes, including district nurses and incontinence advisers.

Social services

Help is provided for people who wish to remain in their own homes, but who cannot manage total care for themselves. Home care assistants will provide many aspects of care of both the individual and their home. Alarm systems may be installed in order that the person can summon help when they need it. Day-care centres provide a place for people to visit during the day, but still return to their own home at night.

For those who are unable to remain in their own homes the social services may provide some residential homes. However, under the National Health Services and Community Care Act 1990, social services can also purchase residential care places for elderly individuals from the private and voluntary sectors.

Housing departments

These departments can provide either sheltered or warden-patrolled housing for elderly people who want to live independently, but need some element of help or supervision.

Voluntary organisations

There are a great many organisations set up to help with the care of elderly people. Some offer direct care, help or advice, while others campaign for elderly people in order to get better provision for them. Examples are Age Concern and Help the Aged.

Private organisations

As the numbers of elderly people have increased, the private sector has emerged as an important supplier of care. The main provision is in the residential care setting, where homes have to be registered with the local social service department. Residential homes may cater for just five residents or they may be very large establishments. If the residents need nursing care, then the homes have to register as nursing homes. Those using the private sector may get some financial help towards the payment of their fees.

To do

List all the services located in your area that help to provide care for elderly people.

People with health problems

Illnesses can be divided into two main categories: physical and psychiatric. Physical illnesses are those that affect the body and the way it functions. Psychiatric conditions affect the way the mind functions and therefore the way that people behave. Illnesses are often classified into disorders of special type or by the body system the disease affects.

Physical

There are three main general types of disorders:

- *infections*, caused by pathogens (germs);
- *cancers*, which have many causes;
- *degenerative disorders*, which may be caused by ageing or other causes.

More details of these conditions can be found in Chapters 8 and 9.

Classification by body systems includes disorders of:

- the *nervous* system, e.g. strokes, Parkinson's disease;
- the *circulatory* system, e.g. varicose veins, angina;
- the *respiratory* system, e.g. asthma, common cold;
- the *digestive* system, e.g. appendicitis, ulcers;
- the *urinary* system, e.g. cystitis, nephritis;
- the *reproductive* system, e.g. fibroids, orchitis;
- the *skin*, e.g. acne, shingles;
- the *skeletal* system, e.g. arthritis, synovitis.

11

Psychiatric

Psychiatric or mental illnesses are divided into two main categories:

- *neuroses*, e.g. anxiety, phobias, depression, hysteria;
- *psychoses*, e.g. manic depression, schizophrenia.

To do

Read through the terms above, and if any are unfamiliar to you check in the glossary at the end of the book or look at other sources.

The services required by people with health problems will depend on the severity of the illness and by the effects the illness has on the body. Many illnesses are minor by nature and people require no outside help, while others may need services at home or to attend other places for treatment or help.

Health

The health services are obviously the main provider of services for people who are sick, but these can be provided either in the home or in other institutions. Doctors or nurses may attend the patient at home or they may attend a health centre. Drugs can be provided on prescription, and other treatments such as chiropody or physiotherapy may be prescribed.

If people are unable to be cared for in their own home, then they may attend clinics, treatment centres or stay in a hospital or hospice.

Hospices

These are often provided by the voluntary sector rather than the NHS, offering specialised care for those who are terminally ill. Some people may remain in this care until they die and others may have short stays to give their family a break, or to try a different type of treatment. The hospice movement has become well known for providing sensitive care, allowing the users to keep their dignity in a relatively pain-free existence. Hospices are often voluntary organisations.

Social services

Social services can provide help to enable people to remain in their own homes through the provision of such services as home care assistants or by having the home adapted to meet the needs of the service user. They can also provide advice on the benefits available.

Private and voluntary organisations

There has been an increase in the amount of private medical care used throughout the UK. Much of this is provided by private medical insurance schemes. The services provided by private health care tend to be for acute rather than chronic cases, for example maternity and surgical cases.

Voluntary groups often act as support groups for people suffering from particular types of disease or illness, e.g. Multiple Sclerosis Society and Cancerlink, while other voluntary groups provide specialist care, e.g. the hospice movement and the Marie Curie Memorial Foundation.

People with disabilities

There is often confusion over the terms handicap and disability. In 1980 the World Health Organisation produced standard international definitions for the following terms.

Impairment: any loss or abnormality of psychological, physiological, or anatomical structure or function.

Disability: any restriction or lack (resulting from an impairment) of ability to perform an activity in the manner or within the range considered normal for a human being.

Handicap: a disadvantage for a given individual, resulting from an impairment or disability, that limits or prevents the fulfilment of a role, depending on age, sex, and social and cultural factors, for that individual.

This means that a disability does not necessarily have to be a handicap if facilities exist to allow for it.

Impairments are usually classified initially into two groups:

- *congenital* – those disabilities which people are born with;
- *acquired* – those disabilities that occur through illness or accidents after birth.

These groups can then be categorised in other ways, depending on the particular disabilities they cause:

- physical;
- psychological;
- both physical and psychological.

To do

List any impairments you can think of, and indicate whether they cause physical, psychological or both types of disability.

Some disabilities can occur both as a result of congenital or acquired impairments, e.g. blindness, deafness and paralysis. Obviously the service required by the individual will depend on the nature and extent of their disability.

Education

In the UK there are special education services provided for those with disabilities. Local schools try to accommodate children with disabilities alongside other children, following the recommendations for integration outlined in the Warnock Report (1978). If for some reason this is not possible, then day or boarding schools can be provided, which cater for children's special needs. Occasionally it may be necessary for a child to receive some education at home.

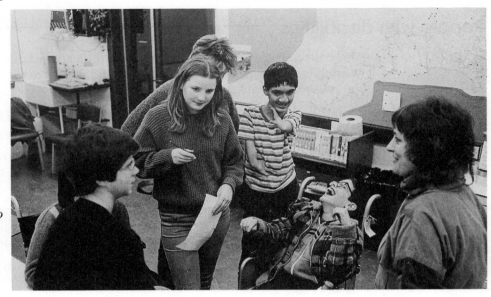

Local schools try to accommodate children with disabilities alongside other children.

These special services extend into further and higher education, and there are also special training workshops provided where people with special needs can learn job skills.

Health

The health service will provide any treatments that may be necessary as they arise. These treatments may include surgery, various types of therapy, such as physiotherapy or occupational therapy, or other forms of care. There is also an advisory service provided for people who think there may be a risk of an inherited disorder being passed on to any children they may have. This service is called genetic counselling.

Preventative measures are also provided, such as immunisation programmes.

Social services

Social services will again provide much in the way of support, either to enable people to remain in their own homes or, if this is not possible, then they may help to provide residential care. One important aspect of care is respite care, where the normal carer can be relieved of their role for short periods of time, and the social services will arrange alternative care. Take, for example, a husband who is caring for his wife who has suffered a stroke, leaving her severely disabled. He has to turn her every four hours during the night, and frequently she disturbs his sleep in between. Social services may arrange for her to be admitted to residential care for a few days, or arrange for someone to stay overnight to provide the care, in order that her husband can sleep through the night.

Again, social services can provide advice about the benefits and services available.

Private and voluntary organisations

For those who can afford to pay for private education or care, limited facilities are available.

Voluntary and charitable organisations provide quite a range of care for people with disabilities and for those who care for them. They may provide residential accommodation, specialist education or training, respite care, support groups and holidays, as well as financing research into the prevention and treatment of many of the disorders. Examples of such organisations include the Spastics Society and the Royal National Institute for the Blind.

Conclusion

Many services are provided for the population of the UK, but even today there are inequalities in both care and those who need it. The poor and some minority groups are those most at risk of suffering illness and disability, and these groups are often unable to get the best out of the services provided. The reasons for this will be discussed in other chapters of the book.

More detailed accounts of the services provided are given in the next two chapters: Chapter 2 which deals with care in the community and Chapter 3 which looks at all aspects of residential care.

Key points

- Most people are cared for by their families in their own homes.
- There are points in everyone's life when their demands on services will be greater than at others.
- The UK provides free services in education, health and social services, to which all are entitled.
- Some services are subsidised and a charge is made on the recipient of that service.
- Some people, such as the poor and some minority groups, are more vulnerable than others.
- The statutory services are often supplemented by the private and voluntary sectors.
- Measures are provided by the services to prevent illness and disability occurring.
- Most services provide both advisory and practical help.

2 Care settings in the community

This chapter will focus on the community, the wide range of settings in which care is provided for service users and the kinds of professional people that you will find working in these settings. The following statutory care providers will be considered:

- social services,
- national health service,
- education,
- housing, and
- probation department,

employing the user groups already defined in Chapter 1.

Keep in mind that, as mentioned in Chapter 1, most caring is provided within the user's own family in the community and it is in the more extreme cases, when the family or other carers are no longer able to cope or do not possess the correct caring skills, that residential or hospital care may be considered as part of the care plan.

Although this chapter will concentrate on the statutory care providers, it is important to remember that the private and voluntary sectors also make an increasing contribution to caring for all kinds of user groups from running day centres for elderly and disabled people to providing advice centres, such as Citizen's Advice Bureaux. In fact, many people would not receive the right degree of care without the support of the voluntary and private services. And, increasingly, the statutory, voluntary and private sectors work together to provide the right package of care for the user. In many instances the statutory services could not provide the right level of care without the support of the voluntary and private sectors.

For example, an adult woman service user with multiple sclerosis in her mid-40s living in her own home, and a wheelchair user, but no longer able to care for herself, might receive help from a range of agencies. As part of her individual care plan the district nurse employed by the national health service might call twice a week to help with bathing and personal hygiene, she might attend the local day centre run by the local multiple sclerosis society twice a week in order to meet her social needs and finally she might pay for help from a private physiotherapist in order to keep her from becoming stiff and pressure sores from developing. This is a 'package of care'.

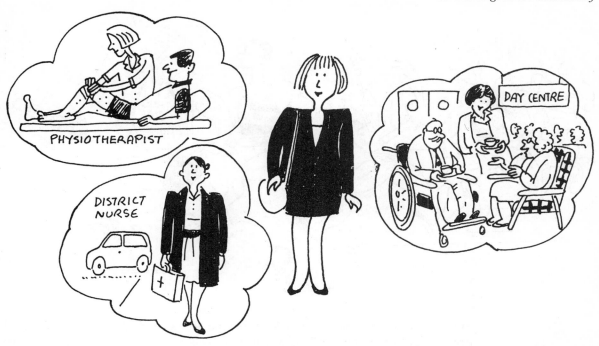

'Here comes that nosy social worker again!'

Community care

As a result of the Griffiths Report on community care, the government is keen to encourage care for all service user groups in the community. The government believes that service users, including elderly people, disabled people, mentally ill people and those with learning difficulties should be able to live in their own homes, wherever possible, with support from outside services to enable them to do this. Residential care should only be considered when a person is no longer able to manage in their own home, even with the support of domiciliary services.

Because of this, a new statute (the National Health Services and Community Care Act 1990) came into force in April 1993. Social service departments have huge new responsibilities for arranging 'community care plans' for service users from the client groups mentioned above. They have responsibility for purchasing services for service users from other organisations in the statutory, voluntary and private sectors. The National Health Service plays a secondary role in this reorganisation.

For example, social services are responsible for putting together a package of care for an elderly person who is discharged from hospital. They first make an assessment of that service user's needs and then if they cannot provide all the services which the elderly person requires in order to remain

17

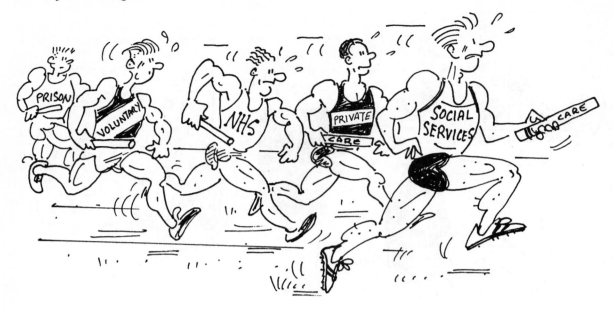

in the community, then they will purchase services from the voluntary and private sectors. Social service departments also have the lead responsibility in making an assessment if a service user is requesting residential care in a rest home or nursing home, but obviously they also need input from the patient's consultant or general practitioner in order to make decisions about the kind of care that is right for that person. Social service departments also have the responsibility of making financial assessments when a service user goes into residential care and for other services. This is a function that they have taken over from the Department of Social Security.

It is important that the service user, and any carers, if the service user agrees, are given a copy of the assessment and involved in the 'package of care', which should be an individual plan to meet the needs of a particular person. If service users feel they are not being treated properly, they can make a complaint to the appropriate person.

We will now go on to consider the role which various statutory departments have to play in caring in the community.

Social service departments

Social services is a local government responsibility aiming to provide advice, counselling and help through a wide range of services for all the categories of people mentioned in Chapter 1. Some people may need help from the department only once in their lives, whereas others may be much more dependent on the services provided by the department.

All social service departments have local offices where clients can drop in for advice, counselling and so on, but social workers will also visit clients in their own homes. Locally-based offices outside large cities usually cover a certain geographical area corresponding to the area covered by the local district council. Their head offices will be based at county hall or, in the case of large cities like Manchester and Birmingham which are metropolitan districts, the main office for social services will be found in the city centre with local offices based in the suburbs.

Local offices

You will find the following professional people based in a local social services office:

- team managers;
- care managers;
- senior social workers;
- social workers;
- social work assistants;
- occupational therapists;
- occupational therapy assistants;
- home care managers and support staff;
- clerical and support staff.

Obviously this list will vary slightly from one area to another, but the basic set-up is that social workers work in teams under a team manager, whose team will be responsible for providing advice and services to a particular client group (see appendix of this book). For example, you may find teams responsible for the following service users:

- children and families;
- elderly people;
- people with a disability;
- mentally ill people;
- people with learning difficulties (including people with severe learning difficulties).

You can either contact social services yourself by visiting the local office or telephoning, or alternatively, and perhaps more likely, you may be referred by somebody else, for example your hospital or general practitioner (GP). Many service users will receive visits from social workers in their own homes. The social worker will then make an assessment of the problem and offer advice, counselling or services which may be appropriate to the problem facing the client.

To do

In pairs consider who else might refer a client to social services and indentify, using the above groups, the kinds of problems different service users might be experiencing.

Service user's own home

Many service users receive a range of services in their own home. For example, elderly people may be recipients of one or more of the following services:

- home help or home care services;
- meals on wheels;
- advice and aids supplied by the occupational therapist;
- advice on benefits;
- support from the social worker.

To do

In pairs or small groups choose one of the service user groups outlined above and research what your local social services department can offer them in terms of advice and services. Prepare a short talk to give to the rest of your group.

Day centres

Most social service departments run day centres for client groups such as elderly people and people with disabilities. Entry to a day centre is usually arranged by a social worker who will have made an assessment, as part of the care plan, of the individual service user's need. Transport is usually provided to and from the centre, and the elderly person may attend one or two days a week, depending on need and the availability of places. A hot lunch is provided. The centre will provide a range of activities for people to become involved in, from painting, bingo, keep fit, budgeting and so on.

However, the aim of most centres, while primarily providing a social function, is to look at the 'whole' person, and consider their physical, psychological and emotional needs as well. For example, a person who has suffered a stroke may have difficulty holding a knife and fork, and can receive help and advice from the occupational therapist. A mentally ill person who is having difficulty budgeting their income could receive advice, support and practical help.

The kinds of personnel you would expect to find in a day centre are:

- a manager;
- care officers and assistants;
- professional staff such as physiotherapists and speech therapists who may be employed on a sessional basis;
- instructors;
- clerical support staff;
- drivers;
- volunteers.

It is important to remember that centres such as these often rely quite heavily on volunteers who may come into work for a day or a few hours, but they are people who give their time freely, carrying out a range of activities, working under the guidance of the professional staff.

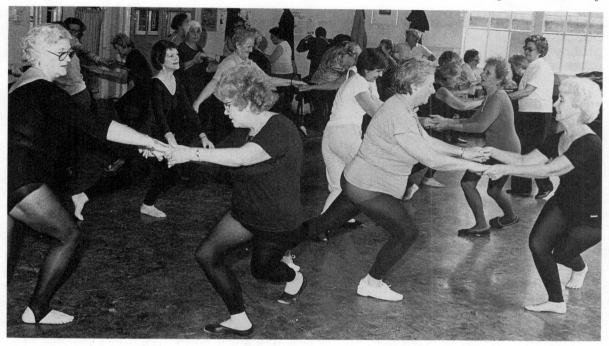

Keep fit for the elderly at Clapham and Battersea Adult Education Institute.

To do

Imagine you are a care assistant in a day centre and you have a new female elderly service user who lives alone and has suffered a stroke. The stroke has affected her left-hand side, particularly her arm. She is left handed. She can walk short distances with the aid of a walking stick and her speech has not been affected. Using the headings of social, physical, psychological and emotional, and working in small groups, think what needs this person might have.

Respite care schemes

These schemes are provided by families in the community who are assessed and approved by the social service department. Respite care schemes can also operate in residential settings. They offer care on a short-term basis, from a few hours to perhaps one or two weeks, in order to give the permanent carer(s) a break from the often stressful occupation of caring full time for someone who is elderly or disabled. The 'respite' families are then paid by social services for the caring they do. The client groups most likely to benefit from this service are:

- elderly people;
- children with a disability;
- young adults or adults with a disability.

Foster or adopt-a-granny scheme

As an alternative to residential care many social service departments operate schemes where an elderly person who can no longer care for themselves in their own home is looked after in a family which has been approved and assessed as competent to care. The families are then paid a weekly fee for the service they perform. This can be a much happier experience for some elderly people who may not want to live in a residential establishment.

Sheltered workshops

Some social service departments are able to offer employment to a range of people who may have a disability, or people who have learning difficulties, on a temporary basis. The idea is that people are employed in a sheltered setting with a view to finding employment in a company locally at a later date. However, people with a disability or learning difficulty will find it harder to get permanent employment in the open market because they may be limited in the kind of work they can do; they may not be able to work at the same pace as other people; or they may find it difficult to relate to other people or not be able to work as an effective team member. Many people with disabilities do find employment in the open market, but it is obviously more difficult and this difficulty is compounded in times of recession when there are large numbers of people who are unemployed.

Sheltered workshops offer those who need it the opportunity to work at a slower pace and to adjust to working with other people as a member of a team. For example, a person who has suffered from mental illness may find it particularly difficult to relate to other people and work as a team member. The kinds of client group that might benefit are:

- mentally ill people;
- young adults with a disability;
- adults with a learning difficulty;
- adults with a disability.

A sheltered workshop is usually run by a manager who has industrial experience and it is the manager's job to obtain contracts from local companies which can be subcontracted to the sheltered workshop.

Training centres

Many people with learning difficulties, especially those with more severe problems, will never be able to live a totally independent life and for many this means that they will not be able to hold down a permanent job in the community. Therefore, many adults with learning difficulties attend training centres which are run by local social service departments.

These centres aim to provide training in social skills, together with the opportunity to become involved in a range of activities, such as improving reading and writing skills for those who are able, and sports activities and outings. Some centres are able to offer opportunities for people to carry out light industrial work and be paid for it.

Most adults attend these centres on a daily basis, and transport is provided to and from the centre. Some adults may be living in residential accommodation in the community provided by the health authority or the social services and attend the centre on a daily basis.

The kinds of professional people who are likely to work in training centres are:

- a manager;
- instructors;
- care assistants;
- clerical support staff.

Volunteers also work in this kind of care setting.

Foster homes

As we have already said, this book does not cover services for children under the age of seven years, but social services are responsible for approving and assessing foster-parents for children and young people of all ages, and this is an extremely important area of their work. The emphasis today is placed on foster care rather than children's homes because it is felt that, wherever possible, the family provides a more caring environment.

Social service departments are responsible for advertising and recruiting their own foster-parents, and they usually run a variety of fostering schemes. It is a lengthy and involved process to be approved as a foster-parent because social services need to be sure that they are recruiting the right kind of people. Once approved foster-parents are paid a weekly rate for the job they are doing and in some instances, if they foster a particularly difficult teenager, they may be paid at a special higher rate.

Adoption

It is worth highlighting the fact that all social services departments also act as adoption agencies. This means that they are responsible for approving adoptive parents, and placing babies and children for adoption.

The difference between adoption and fostering is that when a child is adopted the adoptive parents take on legally and permanently all the legal rights and responsibilities of a natural parent. An adoption order is for life, although once a young person reaches the age of 18 they can, after counselling and advice, try to trace their natural parents if they so desire.

Adoptive homes are a community resource and, as there are fewer and fewer small babies available for adoption, because of the availability of abortion and better contraception information, it is often older children, perhaps with a disability, who are waiting to be adopted.

Intermediate treatment centres

The term intermediate treatment centres is a curious one, used to describe a particular type of 'treatment' which is available to juvenile offenders, both male and female, as an alternative to residential care. When the courts place a supervision order on a young person they can attach intermediate treatment to it as part of the order. So, for example, when a social worker, probation officer or education welfare officer is writing a court report on a young person, aged 14 to 16, they can make a recommendation to the court

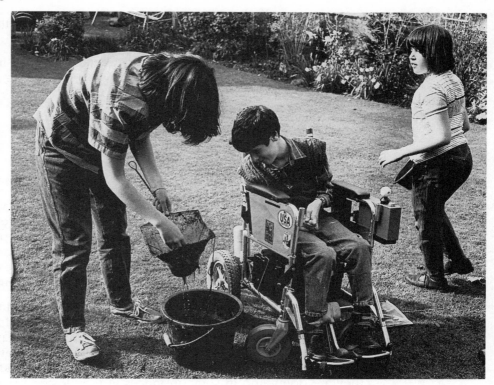

Emphasis is placed on foster care to provide a caring family environment.

that they become involved in intermediate treatment. If the court makes this order the young person then has to attend an IT centre. The kinds of activities that the centre might offer include:

- discussion groups;
- one-to-one counselling;
- practical activities;
- physical activities;
- community placements;
- residential weekends or short holidays.

To do

Social services provide a wide range of services for their users. In small groups choose a care setting in your community and investigate it in more depth. Find out the following by arranging a visit:

- Number of clients/reasons for them being there?
- How are they referred and assessed?
- Admission procedure?
- A typical day?

- What kind of staff are employed there and what qualifications do they need to have?
- What kind of visits and input do they receive from other agencies?

Then plan and prepare a short presentation on your chosen care setting for the rest of the group. If you have access to a video camera you could record your material.

The National Health Service (NHS)

The Department of Health operates the National Health Service through a system of regional and district health authorities (see chart in appendix to this book) in England and Wales. At a local level the district health authority is responsible for:

- assessing local health needs;
- employing staff, both medical and other;
- planning and administering the appropriate services.

If you are considering the NHS and how it functions in the community your starting-off point must be the primary health care team. This term refers to the health service personnel whose job takes them into daily contact with the local community and whose work base is the local GP practice or Health Centre. Most people have some first-hand experience of visiting the doctor and so will be familiar with this kind of care setting.

**GP practice/
health centre**

All service user groups will at some stage in the course of their daily lives come into contact with the primary health care team. Again, demand for services will vary. For example elderly people are obviously going to make a greater demand on the service than young adults.

The general practitioner or family doctor, as they are sometimes known, forms the pivot for the team. The GP is the first person a patient contacts when they are ill, even if it is a minor illness. They can then refer the patient on to the appropriate consultant at the local hospital, or may refer the patient for further tests, e.g. blood tests, or alternatively the GP can refer the patient to community services such as the district nursing service, the midwife, the community psychiatric nurse and so on.

Professional people working from a health centre are as follows:

- general practitioners;
- practice nurses;
- district nurses;
- health visitors;
- midwives;
- community psychiatric nurses;
- counsellors (not in all practices);

- pharmacists (not in all practices, more likely in rural ones);
- practice manager, receptionist and support staff.

Not all surgeries will automatically employ all the personnel listed above. For example not all surgeries will offer a full-time counselling service, but this is becoming more and more common. Alternatively, a local surgery may have an arrangement with the local social services department so a social worker may be available at certain times of the week.

Some surgeries are lucky enough to have other paramedical (supporting) services operating from their surgery and these might include people like:

- chiropodists,
- opticians,
- dentists,

who will also provide a service in the community.

Many GPs are being encouraged by their district health authorities to carry out as many minor operations as they can in their own surgeries, under local anaesthetic, with the assistance of their practice nurses. Examples of this type of operation might be the removal of a cyst or an ingrowing toe-nail. It is cost-effective to do this because it saves referring the patient to a hospital and means more income for the practice.

Patient's own home

All patient groups may be recipients of a variety of health services in their own homes, but there are some patient groups who are more likely to make use of them than others. Examples are:

- elderly people;
- very sick people (all age groups);
- people with disabilities.

For example, a person who is mentally ill may need regular injections and support from the community psychiatric nurse or a physically disabled person who has had a stroke may need help with bathing.

Sometimes, if a patient has been in hospital, and they are returning home, hospital professionals will visit the patient in their own home to ensure that they will be able to cope with the support of various services in the community. Examples of these personnel might be:

- physiotherapist;
- occupational therapist;
- speech therapist;
- chiropodist.

Health clinics

Paramedical services such as:

- speech therapists,
- opticians,

- dentists and
- school nurses

are often based in health clinics.

These professionals will go out and work in the community as well as receiving patients at the clinic. For example, speech therapists will work in special schools and school nurses will be involved in a wide range of illness prevention work in local schools. Examples include advising about injections for German measles or checking children's heads for lice and nits, and telling parents about suitable treatment for this condition.

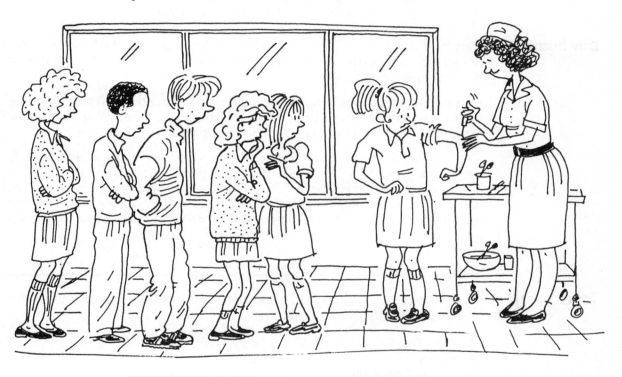

To do

In small groups write letters to health professionals like an occupational therapist, practice nurse, physiotherapist, chiropodist or school nurse and ask them if they would be willing to give a short talk to your group about their role in the community. Telephone the organisation first to find out to whom to address the letter.

There is also a range of services provided by the NHS which are hospital based, yet attended by patients on a daily basis.

Casualty department

If anyone has an accident they can be treated at their local hospital's casualty department. Obviously, depending on the nature of the accident, this may result in further in-patient treatment in hospital or it may mean being assessed and treated in casualty, and being sent home again, or attending the hospital for further treatment on an out-patient basis.

Casualty departments are usually attached to the local district general hospital.

Out-patient clinics

Hospitals provide a wide range of out-patient clinics which people attend on an appointment system to meet a wide range of health needs. A person who has been mentally ill may attend an out-patient clinic, as may someone who has been physically ill or has, perhaps, a broken limb.

Day hospitals

Day hospitals are an increasingly popular development in the health service. Patients attend, as the name suggests, on a daily basis, have their treatment and return home the same day.

As operation times are being cut so it is becoming possible to carry out more and more procedures and operations on this basis. A hernia operation, for example, could be carried out at a day hospital.

The day hospital concept is also extremely successful in the care of elderly people and mentally ill people. Again the patient attends on a daily basis and receives their treatment, but returns to their own home at the end of the day. The advantages for the patient are that they do not have to leave their families and they can continue to receive their support while recovering at home.

To do

In pairs or in small groups investigate more fully the role of one of the following health service personnel:

- occupational therapist;
- speech therapist;
- physiotherapist;
- radiographer;
- pharmacist.

Also, find out what qualifications are needed to enter the above professions and what kind of training they undertake. Report back to the rest of the group.

Education department

It is the responsibility of the local education authority to make educational provision for children who have special needs. Obviously this provision includes children under the age of seven years. Special educational needs covers children with a wide range of disabilities and specific examples include:

- visual;
- hearing;
- autistic;
- epileptic;
- delicate;
- learning difficulties, usually categorised into medium and severe;
- physical;
- emotional.

Under the Education Act 1981, and following the Warnock Report of 1978, these children and young adults are referred to as having 'special educational needs'.

Special schools

Most special schools are controlled and run by the local education authority and there are approximately 2000 of them (in 1993). However, roughly 20 per cent of these are run by voluntary bodies or are private special schools.

The majority of special schools have specially trained teachers and support staff such as physiotherapists and speech therapists, with special facilities to meet the needs of the children and much smaller classes than in an ordinary school. For example, if it is a school that meets the needs of physically disabled children then there will be toilets and washbasins adapted for the children's needs. Some schools have residential facilities as well so that children may board at school during the week and return home to their families at the weekend.

Statementing

As outlined below, some children with less severe special needs will be integrated into ordinary mainstream schools where their educational needs will be met quite successfully. However, in the case of a child who is recognised as having a more severe special educational need, the process of statementing will be activated. A child over the age of two years can be statemented.

Statementing is quite a lengthy process and a formal procedure is laid down under the Education Act 1981. Where possible, parents are to be involved in decisions being made about their child's education, because obviously they may have a lot of information to contribute since they are primarily responsible for the care of their child. During the statementing process reports are received by the local education authority, from the head and teachers at the child's school, from an educational psychologist, from doctors, parents and others from whom parents may have asked for advice to be taken.

Eventually, all this information is gathered together and a formal statement made about which school the child should attend. Parents can appeal if they do not agree with the local authority's decision. A review of that statement, once agreed, must be made every 12 months and the child who is statemented must be reassessed between the ages of 13½ and 14½.

Ordinary schools

Not all children with special needs will attend a special school. Local education authorities (LEAs) are expected, where possible, to integrate such children into the normal schooling system so as they can lead as normal a life as possible. For example, a child with impaired hearing will often be educated in an ordinary school using special equipment such as a phonic ear.

Further and higher education

Further education and tertiary colleges often provide full-time and part-time courses for young adults with special educational needs. The idea is that they should be integrated into the life of the college.

Polytechnics and universities are becoming more aware of students with special educational needs, and more and more special provisions, like ramps, lifts and specially adapted equipment are being provided.

Home tutors

There are a small number of children who are unable to attend school, perhaps because they are ill or experiencing emotional problems, and they can receive tuition at home from teachers who are employed by the local education authority.

To do

In pairs or small groups investigate the availability of special educational provision in your area, both statutory and voluntary. In pairs or small groups arrange to visit your local special schools and give a short report back to the rest of the group.

The education welfare service

Education welfare officers are social workers, based in local schools or LEA offices, who work specifically within the education service. For example, where a child is truanting and not attending school on a regular basis, or where a child is suffering from school phobia or is being bullied it will be the education welfare officer's job to visit the child's family, teachers and so on in order to try to find out what is going wrong. They will then try and work in conjunction with the child and the family to get the young person back to school on a regular basis.

Some larger secondary schools and colleges have full-time counsellors or teachers who are specially trained in dealing with young people's problems. However, they tend not to work in the community and are usually based in a particular school or college.

Housing department

The majority of local authority housing departments provide some rented council accommodation for elderly people and people suffering from some form of disability.

Sheltered housing/ warden serviced accommodation

This rented council accommodation is usually situated in a complex where there are a number of elderly/disabled people living. Each person has their own flat or bedsitter, but there is usually a warden to supervise in case anyone needs help or support. There is an intercom provided between the warden and each flat, and the warden will either visit or call the elderly person on the intercom each day to check that they are all right. In the event of a person needing their GP, for example, the warden will call them in.

Some sheltered housing complexes do not use a warden on site, but have a central control point to which each elderly person's flat is connected by means of pushing a 'panic button' on their ordinary telephone if they are in need of help. The co-ordinator at the other end can then call an ambulance or a mobile warden or make the necessary call in order to summon help for the elderly person.

Probation service

The probation service, which is a local government responsibility, deals mainly with young adults over the age of 17 years and adults who have been convicted of a criminal offence by the courts. The courts have a range of sentencing powers open to them and one choice, instead of sending a person to prison, is to use the probation service. This means that the person serves their 'sentence' in the community. The kinds of sentence the court might choose are:

- a *probation order*, which means the offender is supervised for a period of time laid down by the court;
- a *community service order*, which means that the offender carries out some kind of community work for a specified number of hours laid down by the court, for example painting and decorating a local authority old people's home.

The probation service is also involved in divorce court conciliation work. This means that where a couple with children are divorcing, and there are arguments about which parent the children should live with, the court asks the probation service to prepare a report to help them make the right decisions in the best interests of the children.

The probation office

The probation office is where probation officers are based and their clients visit the office on a regular basis as determined by their individual officer. It is the probation officer's job to assist and befriend their clients, which might mean checking on where they are living, helping them try to find

31

employment if they are out of work and, above all, making sure that the offender does not get into further criminal trouble. Probation officers will visit clients in their own home as well.

It is also the probation officer's job to supervise people who are coming out of prison. Prisoners are released from prison 'on licence' into the community and for a specified period of time, perhaps a year, the ex-prisoner will have to report regularly to a probation officer.

Probation day centres

Many probation services have their own day centres for clients. These day centres provide a range of services from counsellors through to classes aimed at preventing the probationer from offending again.

For example, classes in car mechanics and spraying vehicles may be offered to young people who have been involved in offences such as taking and driving away motor vehicles.

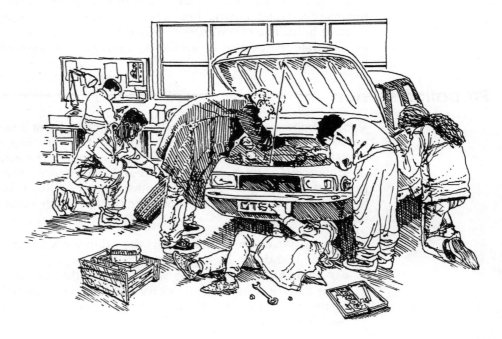

The UK has the highest prison population of any European country and the government is looking at alternative kinds of punishments for more minor offences. This means that in the future more and more offenders will serve their sentences in the community.

Voluntary and private agencies

It is worth mentioning again that it is important not to forget the vast contribution which the voluntary and private sectors make to caring for people in the community, and this applies equally across the whole range of service user groups.

In particular the expansion of private services has been very noticeable during the 1980s, from private health care schemes, alternative medicines and therapies such as chiropractic, herbalism and aromatherapy, through to rest homes and nursing homes for elderly people.

To do

In pairs or small groups choose a local voluntary organisation, arrange to visit them if possible, and write up a short report of the visit. In particular consider the following.

- What range of clients/patients are helped?
- How are they referred?
- What service does the organisation offer?
- Do they employ professionals as well as volunteers?

Key points

- The statutory services providing care in the community are social services, the NHS, education, housing and probation.
- They work in conjunction with the voluntary and private sectors.
- The government is keen to promote a programme of community care for all service users. New laws on community care came into force in April 1993. Social service departments will be the lead agency working in conjunction with statutory, voluntary and private agencies to provide individual care plans (or packages of care) for service users.
- There are a wide range of professionals working in the community.
- In many care practice settings professionals are supported by volunteers.
- Care in the community can often be better for the individual person because, with support, sometimes for a limited period, it maintains a person's dignity, self-respect and independence which they may be in danger of losing if they have to enter residential care.

3 *Residential settings*

As we saw in Chapter 2, there are many agencies providing care in the community. Most of these agencies also provide care in residential settings:

- social services;
- national health service;
- education;
- prison/criminal justice.

It must be stressed again that the voluntary and private sectors play an important part in this provision for the client groups discussed in Chapter 1. The roles of these two important sectors will be discussed in this chapter, together with the most relevant statutory provider.

Residential care is needed when:

- people are no longer able to look after themselves;
- clients are no longer able to be treated or cared for in the community, either independently or supported by community services;
- it is considered that people are not safe living within the community, either for their own or the safety of others.

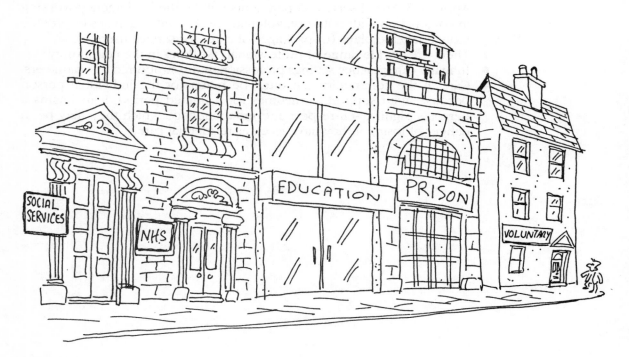

If these admissions are made under the Mental Health Act 1983, the stay may be temporary from up to 72 hours (under section 4), up to 28 days (section 2) or up to 6 months (section 3). Under section 3 this period may be extended for six months more, followed by one year at a time, but after three years it must be reviewed by the Mental Health Review Tribunal.

To do

For many people going into a residential setting means a great upheaval and a dramatic change of lifestyle. Imagine yourself having to leave your present home and go into residential care. Write down a checklist of requirements for your new home. What things do you think you would most miss, and what changes do you think would most affect you? Make some short notes and compare your thoughts with other people in your group.

The Conservative government in the early 1980s was very concerned about the standard of care provided within many residential settings. Following investigations they published a report in 1984 called *Home Life: A Code of Practice for Residential Care*. This report provided advice and guidelines for people running and working in residential homes. Some of the main points they made centred on trying to allow as much independence as possible and enabling clients to retain their privacy and dignity.

Some of the main principles laid down for the rights of residents included:

- *fulfilment* – achieving their full potential;
- *dignity* – preservation of self-respect;
- *autonomy* – right to self-determination;
- *individuality* – individual needs and preferences met;
- *esteem* – importance placed on their qualities and experiences;
- *quality of experience* – provision of a wide range of normal activities;
- *emotional needs* – normal opportunities for emotional expression;
- *risk and choice* – to take risks and make choices, as long as other people are not endangered.

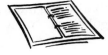

Case study

Mrs Whittaker was widowed 2 years ago, after being married for 52 years. Since then she has lived on her own, with support from her married son and married daughter, as well as a home care assistant and meals on wheels. However, she is now severely incapacitated by osteo-arthritis and she feels she needs to move into residential care. Her family are unable to provide a home for her, because of their own children, and her social worker has found a place for her in a residential home. She is still anxious to maintain some independence, and although she is aware of her own physical limitations she has retained her full psychological capacities.

To do

As a care assistant in the residential home accepting Mrs Whittaker, how could you try to ensure that her rights (as outlined on page 35) are met? Make notes on your suggestions, giving practical examples, and discuss these with others either in your study or work group. If you are a member of a study group, simulate the admission procedure of this resident, with one of you taking the role of Mrs Whittaker and others playing the various staff and other residents.

These principles should form a guideline for the provision of all types of residential care, regardless of the client group. We are now going to examine how the different agencies, where applicable, provide care for the client groups discussed in Chapter 1.

Social services

Children

When children are not able to be cared for by their own family within the family home there are several options open to social services. Research findings, reported in 1990, gave the use of these options as:

Fostering	48%
Community homes	22%
Guardian, relative, friend	17%
Lodgings, flat	10%
Voluntary homes	3%

Adoption and fostering were discussed in Chapter 2, in this section we will look at other forms of residential care.

Residential homes

Most residential homes are now provided by the local authority, but some voluntary homes still exist, for example National Children's Homes. Voluntary children's homes were offering about 12 000 places in 1992. Most residential homes are small, typically housing about ten children under the care of house parents, with the main aim being to provide a close, secure and loving atmosphere. In south-east England a small number of private residential homes exist, which are run on a profit-making basis. These, and the voluntary homes, have to be registered with the local authority and must be open to inspection, as well as complying with certain regulations, under the Children Act 1989.

Adults

Social services (together with housing departments) have responsibilities for two main categories of adults, namely single mothers and homeless families.

In many local authorities, these services are provided by the housing department rather than by social services.

Single mothers

Single mothers may be catered for in mother-and-baby homes, of which there are about 150 in the UK. Some of these are provided by social services,

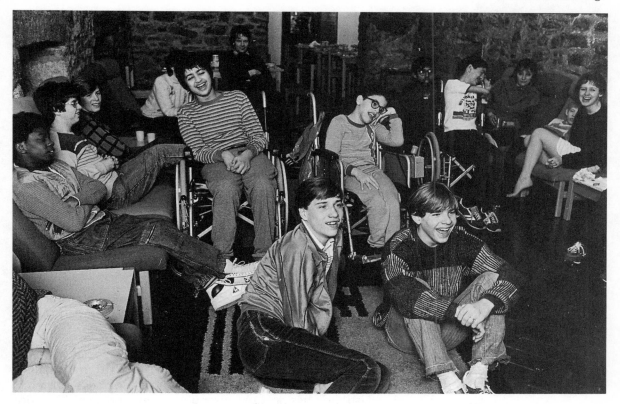

When children are not able to be cared for by their own family within the family home, one of the options available to the social services is residential homes.

but most of them are run by voluntary organisations, often subsidised by local authorities. These usually provide care for about six weeks before and after the birth of the baby.

Homeless families

The problem of homeless families has increased over the years, as local authorities do not have enough accommodation to house all the homeless people they come across. About 40 per cent of people become homeless when families or friends are no longer able or willing to offer accommodation, 20 per cent are made homeless through marriage or partnership breakdown and 14 per cent as a consequence of non-payment of mortgages or rent.

Accommodation offered by local authorities includes:

- hostels;
- family units in council property;
- hotels or guest houses.

The service is supplemented by many voluntary organisations, such as the Salvation Army; and there are also about 2650 housing associations providing accommodation for homeless people, as well as creating permanent accommodation for renting or co-ownership.

Local authorities also sponsor some housing advisory and aid centres which give advice and information on tenancy rights etc., in an attempt to prevent families from becoming homeless. Many voluntary groups such as SHAC (Shelter Housing Aid Centre) also provide a similar service.

Elderly and disabled people

In Chapter 2 we discussed the many different types of provision that are made in order to keep elderly people, and those with disabilities, in the community, and in fact only about 2.5 per cent of elderly people currently (1993) live in residential homes. Homes for these client groups are provided for by local authorities through the social services department, but over half are catered for in private or voluntary homes. From 1993 social service departments will be able to purchase places for individuals within the private sector in order to supplement their own provision. These will be for people who cannot afford the fees charged in the private sector, but have been assessed as requiring residential care. The modern trend is to provide care in smaller units, rarely with more than 40 residents, and many being much smaller.

For some groups of people with learning difficulties residential accommodation is provided by hostels that are often jointly funded by the NHS and social services.

All private and voluntary homes have to be registered with social services, and most social service departments would have a separate unit dealing with these registrations. Since 1984 and the introduction of the Registered Homes Act, this registration has become compulsory, and the local authority should carry out annual inspections to ensure that satisfactory standards are being met. Many of the intentions behind the Act are based on the findings of the *Home Life Report* of 1984, mentioned previously. If the residents are in need of nursing care then the homes have to be registered as nursing homes and must employ suitable numbers of qualified nursing staff in order to provide sufficient care. Staff of residential homes are not all qualified, but the person in charge should either be a registered nurse or a qualified social worker. Currently owners of residential homes are being encouraged to train all their staff. It is hoped that the new national vocational qualifications (NVQs) will provide these staff with nationally recognised qualifications.

As already stated people can get some financial support if they cannot afford the full cost from their own financial resources. Under the NHS and Community Care Act 1990 this will be provided as follows.

From 1993 all existing residents in homes will be protected and continue to receive Department of Social Security support if they were already in receipt of benefits, or if they were in a registered (or equivalent) home and their own resources run out. All new or prospective residents in independent or private sector homes will need to be assessed professionally and financially if they do not pay from private resources. The fee will be paid in full by the social service department, and a contract made between the home and the local authority.

To do

Think of the needs of *either* a teenager *or* an elderly person going into residential care (using your work place experiences if possible). If you were going to design a small home for 14 residents what features would you include to try to ensure that these needs can be met?

National Health Service

The NHS mainly provides services for those people who have health problems, although the patients may come from any of the client categories listed in Chapter 1. These health problems may be caused through illness or through injuries or trauma.

There are two main types of hospitals in the NHS, these being:

- general hospitals;
- psychiatric hospitals.

Hospitals are administered by regional health authorities, through locally administered district health authorities, who advise on local needs and run the local services. General hospitals provide services for those who need treatment for physical conditions; psychiatric hospitals for those clients with psychological problems.

Since 1991 the government has allowed some hospitals to become self-governing trusts, which means that they can charge the district health authority for its services. This will alter the structure and management from the traditional model shown below. As the number of trusts increases then the district health authorities will become purchasers of services, rather than manager and provider.

In 1990 there were approximately 2500 hospitals in England and Wales, some of them offering specialist services only. For example, there are 200 maternity hospitals, 300 for mentally disordered and 300 for long-stay patients. Between them they offer about 400 000 beds, giving treatment to about 7 million patients per year. One of the biggest changes in in-patient treatment over the years is the length of stay: in 1966 the average length of stay was 18.6 days, compared with 8 in 1984.

In addition to the NHS, there are an increasing number of private hospitals, usually managed by a few large companies and often linked to private health insurance firms. About 70 per cent of admissions to private hospitals are covered by insurance, the two main companies being BUPA (British United Provident Association) and PPP (Private Patients Plan). These hospitals usually provide for acute care rather than for chronic or long-term illnesses or conditions. In 1990 there were about 150 hospitals, plus nursing homes in the private sector, providing 7200 beds and 300 000 treatments a year.

NHS hospitals provide treatment for all types of illness, and although some hospitals may specialise in one type of care, general hospitals usually admit

Structure of NHS Hospital Service

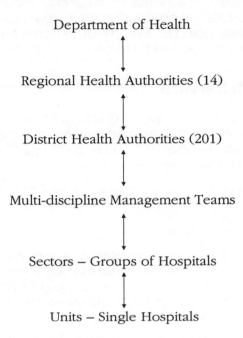

Department of Health

↕

Regional Health Authorities (14)

↕

District Health Authorities (201)

↕

Multi-discipline Management Teams

↕

Sectors – Groups of Hospitals

↕

Units – Single Hospitals

anyone from their district or area who needs care. Some expensive or very specialised types of treatment may not be offered by every hospital in a region, but only by one or two, in order to save duplication of resources. Examples of these types of treatment are renal or kidney dialysis, transplants, burns, cardiac surgery, and plastic or cosmetic surgery.

To do

Either as individuals or in a group, find out how many hospitals there are in your area. List the types of services they offer, and try and find out where patients have to go for specialist treatments that are not provided by your local hospital.

The types of beds or services offered by the NHS are classified under seven headings:

- surgical;
- medical;
- chronic sick and care of elderly people;
- mental handicap;
- mental illness;
- maternity;
- other.

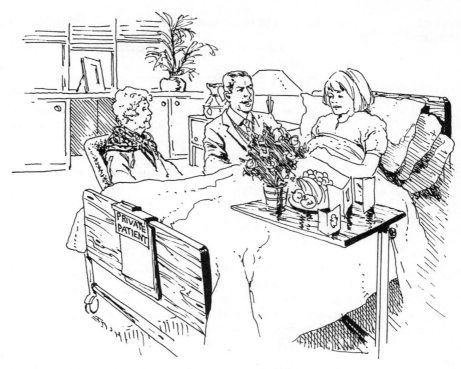

The division of beds within the NHS is shown by the pie chart below.

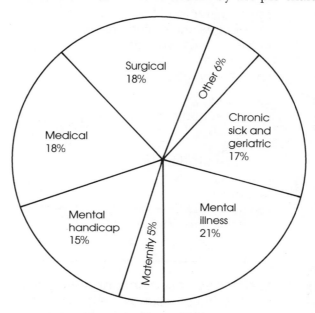

Hospital beds, England and Wales, 1987 (350 000)

From T. Byrne and C. Padfield, *Social Services*

Types of treatment

Treatment in general hospitals can usually be divided into:

- *diagnostic* – carrying out examinations and tests in order to diagnose the condition;
- *surgical* – carrying out surgery to correct a condition, either through removal of diseased tissue or to correct a malfunction or malformation;
- *medical* – usually either through chemotherapy, treatment with drugs, or through other therapies, such as physio, speech, occupational or radio-therapy.

Staffing

The NHS is one of the UK's biggest employers, employing people within the following categories.

Medical

consultants,
registrars,
house doctors.

Nursing

registered general nurses,
registered mental nurses,
registered mental handicap nurses,
registered sick children's nurses,
state certified midwives,
state enrolled nurses (this grade is being phased out).

These different types of qualified nurses are all paid on a graded structure, dependent upon their qualifications and responsibilities.

Paramedics

physiotherapists,
radiologists and radiotherapists,
occupational therapists,
pharmacists,
speech therapists.

Support staff

laboratory,
health support workers (replacing the therapy helpers and nursing assistants),
catering,
clerical and administration,
cleaning,
laundry,
estates and maintenance,
portering and driving.

To do

Imagine you are a patient, having suffered a stroke, or if you have been a patient, use your own experience. Using the list of staff above, think who may be involved with your stay in hospital and write a short summary of the role they might play.

Admission to hospital

There are normally two routes of entry to hospital as an in-patient, these are:

- emergency admission;
- 'cold' or booked admission.

Emergency admission

If someone is taken ill suddenly, or has an accident which necessitates treatment as an in-patient, they are usually admitted through the casualty unit or department.

Patients may go themselves or their relatives may take them there, they may be brought in by ambulance or referred there by their own doctor or general practitioner. In most cases a bed is made available, although there may sometimes by a delay before a bed can be found. If the hospital staff think it desirable the patient may be transferred to a specialist unit in another hospital.

Booked or 'cold' admission

This means that patients are admitted to hospital for treatment of a condition that is not an emergency. Usually these patients will have been seen by a hospital doctor at an out-patient department or clinic, and if the doctor thinks in-patient treatment is necessary the person is placed on the waiting list, then called for admission when their turn comes. The waiting lists are prioritised, with life-threatening conditions taking priority over other conditions that may still be causing a person a great deal of distress and pain.

These waiting lists are the subject of much debate and criticism, and the newly introduced Health Charter indicates that no one should have to wait more than two years for a bed. However, in reality, this is still often not the case. It is estimated (1993) that at any one time there are 700 000 people on the waiting list for all hospitals in England and Wales.

Some general practitioners now have the option of sending their patients elsewhere for treatment, if a hospital other than their own district hospital can admit the patient more quickly. Alternatively, the patients themselves may decide that they would prefer to pay for their own treatment through the private sector, rather than wait for treatment through the NHS.

A pregnant women is booked into a maternity unit and then admitted as an emergency when she goes into labour, unless she has decided on a home birth.

To do

Draw up two lists: one giving ten reasons for emergency admission; the other giving ten reasons for booked admissions. Prioritise your booked admissions, giving reasons for your decisions. Discuss your decisions with your group and see if they agree with your reasons.

As we have already seen, most in-patients have a short stay in hospital, and once well enough they are discharged, to be cared for by the community services as described in Chapter 2. However, for some patients long-term hospital care is needed, especially for some psychiatric conditions.

Specific client groups

Elderly people

Provision for the care of elderly people is one of the priority areas in the UK, because of the large numbers in the population. It has been estimated that the average person goes into hospital once every 10 years, but for those over the age of 75 the frequency doubles. While only 2 per cent of elderly people are in hospital, they occupy over half the beds, with those over 75 taking one-third of all beds. District general hospitals have special units with a range of diagnostic and treatment facilities. Their aim is to treat and rehabilitate elderly patients in order that they may return to the community as soon as possible. It is hoped that under the new care in the community provisions, many more facilities will be provided for elderly people to be cared for at home or in residential homes, rather than in hospital settings.

Psychiatric patients

In 1988 there were about 103 000 people in psychiatric hospitals, of these 65 000 were described as being mentally ill, while 37 000 were there because of a mental disability. Most of these patients are in hospital as voluntary patients, but about 10 per cent (20 000) of mentally ill admissions and under 5 per cent (600) of mentally disabled admissions are detained by force of law, under the Mental Health Act 1983.

Most of the patients receiving long-term residential care are either those with severe handicaps or those suffering from psychotic rather than neurotic illnesses. Today the treatment these patients undergo falls into two main categories:

- *chemotherapy* (in the general sense of drug treatments) – these may control the condition or help to cure it;
- *psychotherapy,* either individual or group – this attempts to enable patients to overcome their problems and be rehabilitated for life in the community.

For mentally disabled patients two other forms of therapy are usually involved:

- *occupational therapy* – rehabilitation through constructive and purposeful activity;
- *industrial therapy* – based on semi-industrial production lines in sheltered workshops or in adult training centres (see Chapter 2).

In 1981 the DHSS estimated that about 15 000 mentally disabled people (including 2000 children) and 5000 mentally ill people in psychiatric hospitals could be cared for in the community if suitable places could be found for them. It is hoped that, under the National Health Services and Community Care Act 1990, the health and social services will together develop care in the community as a joint approach that will enable a great many more current in-patients to be discharged into appropriate community settings.

Education

As we saw in Chapter 2, most education services are provided within the community, with children attending on a daily basis. However, some residential or boarding schools do exist, but many of these are in the private sector. The state sector may provide some residential places in community schools if part of the catchment area is very rural or if there are transport problems.

Private sector

In the UK there is a long-established tradition of sending children to fee-paying or independent schools, including public schools (about 300 in 1993). The private sector provides for about 6 per cent of the school population, over half a million pupils, through 2500 schools. Many of these schools are boarding or residential. They include preparatory schools which cater for children aged 8 to 13. Some schools offer an assisted places scheme, where children of less well-off parents have their school fees remitted by the 230 independent schools in the scheme.

Others who get help with residential school provision are those whose parents are in the armed forces, or otherwise working abroad. This help is provided by the employer or perhaps by the local education authority, who will also occasionally pay for this kind of assistance where home circumstances are unsatisfactory for some reason.

Higher education

Students attending universities, colleges or institutes of higher education often need to be in residential accommodation. This may be in college halls of residence or in private lodgings. The students themselves, or their parents, are expected to pay these costs, although some may get grants or loans.

Special schools

Special schools are provided for those pupils with mental or physical disabilities. Following the Warnock Report in 1978 and the Education Act 1981, these children are known as children having 'special educational needs'. If they cannot be integrated into ordinary schools, it may become necessary to provide special schools for them and some of these will have residential facilities. Some of these may be provided by local education authorities, but others are set up by charities or voluntary groups, such as the Autistic Society and the Spastics Society.

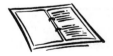

Case study

Two cousins, both aged 11, are about to start their secondary education. Neither of them has any brothers or sisters. One of them, Sarah, was born with a severe sight impairment, and is registered partially sighted; she has so far been educated at home, as the nearest junior school was 14 miles away. Her cousin, Mark, suffers from muscular dystrophy, which has meant that for the last three years he has been using a wheelchair for mobility. He has attended his local junior school, but the local secondary school is ten miles away, and is a two-storey building. Together the

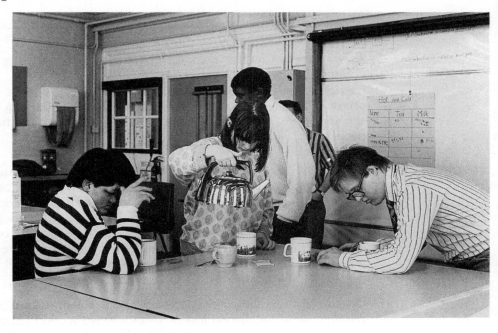

Students from a special school cooking at Islington Sixth Form Centre.

children and their parents have to decide on which option to choose for secondary education. Should they be educated at home, their local secondary school, an ordinary shool with residential accommodation or special boarding schools equipped to cater for their special needs?

To do

Draw up tables for both Sarah and Mark, showing the advantages and disadvantages of each method of education. From your tables try to decide which you think are the best options for these two children, giving your reasons.

Prison services

The law says that people have to reach a certain age before they are criminally responsible. The guidelines are:

- *under 10* – not criminally liable;
- *between 10 and 14* – under the age of criminal responsibility, but liable to care proceedings;
- *over 14 and under 17* – *fully liable for criminal acts.*

Young people between the ages of 16 and 18 are tried in Youth Courts, which under the Children Act 1989 replaced the Juvenile Courts. They will be sentenced in the same way as adults in Magistrates' or Crown Courts. For serious offences young people may be referred to either of these courts.

Young people found quilty of committing a crime may be punished by a variety of means, including those discussed in Chapter 2. However, they may also be sentenced to serve a custodial or semi-custodial sentence.

Custodial sentences include:

- imprisonment;
- hospital order;
- youth custody centre;
- community homes;
- care orders.

Imprisonment Adult offenders may be sent to one of HM prisons, some of which are 'closed', where prisoners have no access to the outside, while others are 'open', where prisoners are allowed a relative freedom, having more contact with the outside, often working outside the prison grounds. In line with current government thinking, some of the prison services are now being privatised, although having to operate within the legal framework and limitations. Broadmoor Mental Hospital and Ashworth Hospital in Liverpool,

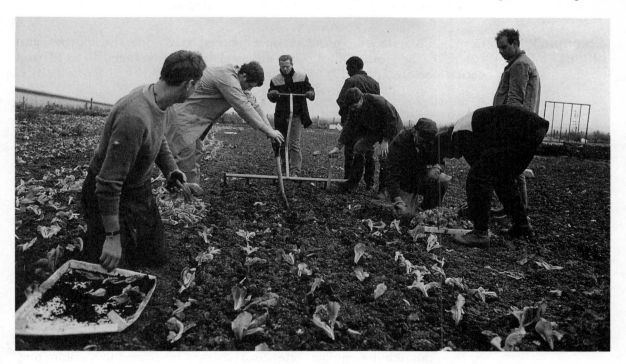

Inmates working on the prison farm at Standford Hill Open Prison, Isle of Sheppey.

known as special hospitals, are allocated for those suffering from insanity or those to be detained 'during HM pleasure' (for an indefinite period). A Crown Court can award any sentence that can be imposed by law, but a Magistrates' Court may not impose a sentence of more than six months for any one offence.

Hospital order

A hospital order may be imposed on an offender who is suffering from:

- mental disorder;
- severe mental impairment;
- mental impairment;
- psychopathic disorder.

Evidence as to the disorder or impairment has to be provided by two doctors, and the purpose of the order is to enable the offender to be detained compulsorily, as long as it is in the offender's and the public's interest. Treatment will be given and the case reviewed from time to time by the managers of the hospital, and the patient can appeal against detention to the Mental Health Review Tribunal.

Youth custody centres

Youth custody centres are for young offenders aged between 17 and 21 years, and they replaced the 'Borstal' system. The sentence may only be passed by a Crown Court, may not exceed three years and must be for a determined period. The emphasis is on training and rehabilitation.

Community homes

Community homes are provided on a regional basis under the approval and control of the Home Office. They are used for children (aged 10 to 14) and young persons (14 to 17) for the purpose of:

- remand,
- correction, and
- care,

where there has been a serious offence. They vary in the form of treatment, accommodation and restriction they offer. Some provide education.

Care orders

Care orders are made by a court committing an offender to the care of a local authority. Orders may also be made on children or young people who are the subject of 'significant harm' at the hands of parents, e.g. physical or sexual abuse. Orders may be made where a child or young person is in need of:

- care,
- protection, and
- control,

or has committed a criminal offence. They may be placed in a community home, foster home, or subject to a hospital order or a guardianship order.

Summary

There has been much publicity about the problem of overcrowding in British prisons, and the conditions within them. Many people argue that custodial sentences should only be used when either the public or the individual is at serious risk, and that for those who are given a custodial sentence, rehabilitation back into the community should be the main principle behind their sentence.

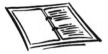

—————————————— **Case study** ——————————————

Mike, a 14-year-old, has been caught shop-lifting for the first time. He was with a group of other young people:

- Sam, 16 years, who has admitted shop-lifting on six previous occasions;
- Angie, 17 years, this is her third time of committing the offence;
- Sarah, 17 years, her first offence;
- Tracey who is 24 and thought to be the ringleader. Tracy has been convicted on two previous occasions. The first time she was given a caution and the second time, at the age of 19, she admitted to ten offences and was put on probation for two years.

To do

What do you think should happen to the young people listed above? Which do you think would be the better options for them? Give reasons for your decisions based on the information provided in this chapter and Chapter 2.

 Key points ——————————————

- Most people only enter residential care for two main reasons:
  – they can no longer be looked after in the community either by themselves or with help from the community services; or
  – it is no longer safe for them or for the public if they remain within the community.
- The main aim of residential care is that, wherever possible, people should be rehabilitated in order that they may return to the community.
- People in residential care should be allowed to retain as much independence as possible, and at all times should be able to retain their dignity and rights to privacy.
- The carers should aim to provide for the meeting of the full range of the residents' needs – physical, intellectual, emotional and social.
- The private and voluntary sectors are very important providers of residential care, although the state may help to pay for the costs of these provisions.
- Only a very small proportion of the population are cared for in residential settings, with elderly people and disabled people forming the largest single client groups. However, only 2.5 per cent of the elderly population live in residential homes.

- Under the Community Care Act 1990, implemented in 1993, it is hoped that the health and social services departments will work closely together to develop community care approaches that will enable more people to remain in the community rather than in residential care.
- Great progress has already been made in the care of children, with most children now being cared for in foster homes or being adopted, meaning that fewer children are in children's homes.
- One of the main aims of custodial care for offenders is to rehabilitate them for life in the community. However, a high percentage of people who have served a custodial sentence offend again.
- The length of stay for the average patient in a NHS hospital bed was reduced from 18.6 days in 1966 to 8 days in 1984.

4 *The individual and society*

In 1986, the then prime minister Margaret Thatcher made a controversial statement that 'there is no such thing as society, there are only individuals'. At the time this viewpoint aroused great debate because it implied that the communities in which we live had no relevance, that between the family and the state, as represented by government, there was a void. Those involved in the care sector might have been particularly alarmed as the concept of *community* care is central to policy at the present time. This is the political dimension to what Mrs Thatcher said, since it was intended to support her views about reducing the level of state and local government intervention in the provision of public services such as schools and hospitals. However, her remarks also reflected a more basic issue about the relative importance of heredity or environment in the development of people from childhood to adulthood. It is reasonable to assume that Mrs Thatcher would believe in the heredity argument, that the individual's genetic blueprint creates the intelligence, personality and physical characteristics which are capable of overcoming the events that are experienced in life. She was born into a fairly modest family and grew up to dominate British and world politics for over a decade. It is not therefore surprising that she made the comments she did. On the other hand, many would argue that the *circumstances* a child is born into will determine the level of achievement and success they have.

The theme of this chapter, then, is to investigate the relationships between the individual, their family, the community and larger society around them. In so doing we will highlight the reasons why some categories of people are more likely to come into care, or need the support of the welfare state as outlined in Chapter 3. We will concentrate on the following aspects of what is a very large and complex area of study:

- an introduction to the concept of *socialisation* and the agencies of socialisation;
- an introduction to the key factors in the socioeconomic environment which affect the lives of individuals at various ages and stages in their development;
- a description and analysis of different types of family life and the influence that each may have;
- an outline of the contribution to development that the other agencies of socialisation make.

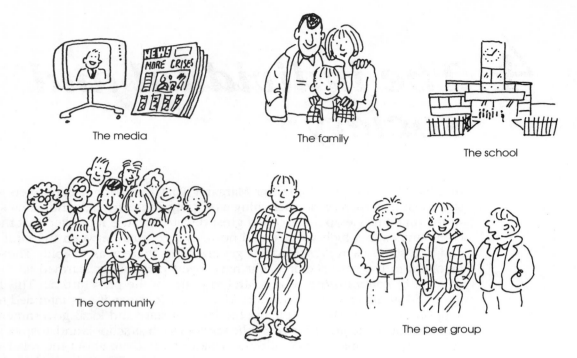

The socialisation process

The media

The family

The school

The community

The peer group

These areas concentrate on a *sociological* view of the individual; sociology is the study of human behaviour by analysing the effects of social interaction and social systems. In effect this means that we will be looking at the environmental factors which influence child development. In Chapters 8 and 9 the physical and psychological factors associated with heredity will be looked at in more detail. There is no conclusive evidence on either side of the debate to prove that one or the other is the most correct, and this chapter will take the view that both sets of factors have to be taken into account.

Socialisation

Socialisation refers to the process of preparing the individual for the appropriate performance of their roles and duties in adult life. It is a lifelong process of learning and adaptation which involves the acquiring of knowledge and skills, the acceptance of the rules within society which govern our behaviour and the tailoring of the personality to these varying requirements. These social and moral rules can differ from society to society, and within societies, and are defined by sociologists as being part of our *culture*. The sociological definition of culture is very broad and includes all aspects of life within a given community, from their religion to what they eat for breakfast, rather than just referring to art or music. This complex web of knowledge and beliefs is passed on by various means and through different agencies. There are four main agencies of socialisation:

- the family;
- the school and educational system in general;
- the mass media – television, radio, the press, cinema etc.;
- the peer group – those friends who are important in both adolescence and later life.

Primary and secondary socialisation

Of these four aspects the family is by far the most important and will be the focus of much of the discussion in this chapter. The nurturing and development of the child within the family setting is referred to as *primary socialisation.* The influence of the other aspects does not normally occur until after about five years of age; their role is defined in the process of *secondary socialisation.* The key role of the family is to ensure that the child, in the crucial first five years, is allowed to grow and develop in an atmosphere of love and security. When a child is born it has a blueprint of physical, intellectual and personality characteristics which are raw and underdeveloped. During these early years it is the parents, or other immediate carers if not the parents, who create the bond with the infant and will shape these characteristics. There is much evidence to show that these innate abilities can be arrested or stimulated by the quality of parent – child interactions. The sociological view talks about the parents as role models. As the child gets older his or her parents will come to represent all adults in society and the child will be deeply influenced by their behaviour both towards their children and to one another. For example, children who have been abused or received inadequate parenting may grow up to be abusing or inadequate parents themselves.

The distinction between primary and secondary socialisation is, however, becoming blurred. This is because the family unit has weakened dramatically over the last few decades, and many difference child-rearing arrangements are now present as substitutes for the traditional family environment.

When we referred earlier to 'communities' the idea of a town, village or neighboorhood may have come to mind, and these communities contain families who will be very different in their lifestyles and beliefs. This is important because 'community' can sometimes refer to groups of people who think or behave the same way, sometimes at odds with more generally held views. They possess a *sub-culture* which, while being similar in many ways to mainstream culture, nevertheless have customs, rules or moral beliefs which are quite different and set them apart. Two good examples of these types of sub-culture are Jehovah's Witnesses and gypsies. Children growing up in these types of families can therefore experience quite conflicting information about what is acceptable or unacceptable behaviour. However, evidence suggests that the influence of the family will nearly always dominate that of the school, the television or the peer group.

To do

Take two different examples of sub-cultures within British society. Describe as many features of their belief systems which are different to the mainstream as you can. Finally, describe briefly, through the eyes of the children from those families, what difficulty or conflict might occur between family life and other aspects of life – in school, among peers etc.

Main influences upon socialisation

It will be clear from the examples that you have used that the socialisation process does not happen in a uniform way: for each individual the arrangement of life circumstances – type of family, social background, type of community and so on – will affect them differently. It is important to take account of these influences which cut across the path through childhood and adolescence into adulthood and, finally, old age. These influences can be listed under the following headings:

- socioeconomic groups;
- gender; and
- race.

Socioeconomic groups

Many sociological studies have been devoted to the investigation of the effects of socioeconomic groups or 'class' on life chances. Class is accepted as being a powerful influence in British life, and although the class lines are far less obvious today compared to the first half of the 20th century, they are still present and have been shown to determine the life chances of children, especially those born into the highest and lowest classes. It is not appropriate here to discuss the best way of defining class, so the government's own scale will be used. This identifies six socioeconomic categories:

A – often referred to as upper class, including those with unearned income, and senior jobs in politics, industry, commerce etc.;

B and *C1* – often referred to as middle class, and includes all white-collar workers, professionals such as teachers, social workers and accountants etc.;

C2, *D* and *E* – often referred to as working class, and including everyone who has a manual job, skilled to unskilled, and the unemployed.

To do

What social group or class do you belong to? Go to the library and find out where the Registrar-General's classification can be found. Where would your family be put? Does it matter? List ten aspects of your lifesyle which you think would be very different if you had been born into another class group. Do you think your social group has advantaged, disadvantaged or not affected your chances in life?

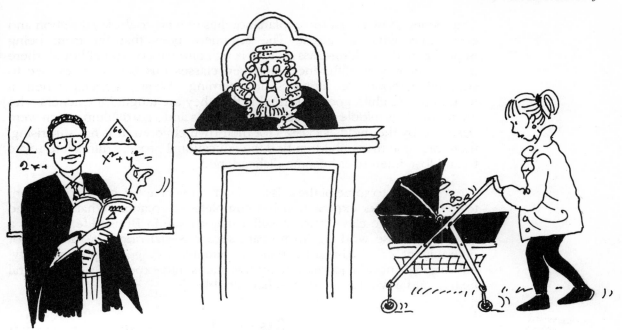

A classless society?

Although it is possible to make direct comparisons between class and wealth, this is a very difficult area. There are many people who are called middle class who are far less prosperous than people from the traditional working class. Today, it is possible for the working class man or woman to buy the trappings of an upper-class lifestyle, by sending their children to public schools for instance. In fact, the strongest area of continuing influence of class outside the family is probably in education, where children from working-class backgrounds have traditionally found progress more difficult to achieve than their middle-class counterparts. This, in turn, affects their ability to obtain high status and high-income jobs after full-time education has finished. A study in the 1960s showed that 7 year olds with similar IQ measurements at that age got significantly different GCE results at 16, and that success was closely correlated to class background. Another more recent study showed that children from social groups A and B are 17 times more likely to go to university than children from classes D and E.

What are the reasons for this? There are two main types of explanation. One is to do with the quality of home life and argues that children from working-class backgrounds suffer from *cultural deprivation* when compared to middle or upper-class children. Working-class children are more likely to have poor or crowded housing, a poor diet, less money to spend on activities, have fewer books, watch more TV and have less 'quality' conversation with parents and other family members, and so on. This lifestyle is said to have a negative influence on the child's intellectual potential and their attitude to education and learning.

The second view is that the explanation lies in who controls education and determines what is taught. The argument goes that far from being impoverished, working-class culture is rich and varied, and although there may be economic differences between classes this has no relevance to parental support or attitudes to learning. What happens when a working-class child goes to school is that they are taught by teachers who are themselves middle class, according to rules and a curriculum which were designed by the middles classes for their own children. It is not surprising, therefore, that many children find the educational process difficult to relate to and lose interest or become disheartened.

We will return to some of these issues later in the chapter, but it is important to say that neither explanation has complete acceptance. What is beyond doubt is that the class factor is still a major issue in British life, and, as a result, for those working in the care sector. Social origin is still a major determinant of child-rearing patterns, family size, geographic mobility, educational success, job and economic status, life expectancy and general health, and a whole variety of other variables.

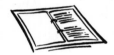

Case study

In a famous TV series called '7 Up' charting the lives of a group of seven year olds, a clear demonstration of the importance of class was given. The first of the series, in 1964, was followed at seven-year intervals to the point in 1992 when the studies were 35. We saw three boys from an exclusive preparatory school who were able to predict which school and university (Oxbridge) that they would be going to at 11 and 18 respectively. They got the predictions almost exactly right. On the other hand we saw children from working-class backgrounds whose horizons were no further than the next week. In likes and dislikes, in language and accent, in expectations and attitudes, these programmes showed a gulf between the different children. Interestingly, however, by the time that they had reached 35 some of those differences were less evident, and for the most part they were not keen to highlight the inequalities and the class divide between them.

Gender

One major distinction within the socialisation process is the experience of growing up as a male or as a female. The changes in the roles that women perform have been dramatic since the Second World War, and this has both a cause and effect relationship with how girls are raised. The key changes have been:

- an increase in the numbers of women who are following careers;
- an increase in the sharing of family responsibilities between partners, rather than the role being clearly segregated on gender lines;
- smaller families with fewer children and fewer family ties;
- the increase in the use of alternative forms of child rearing other than by the birth parents on their own;

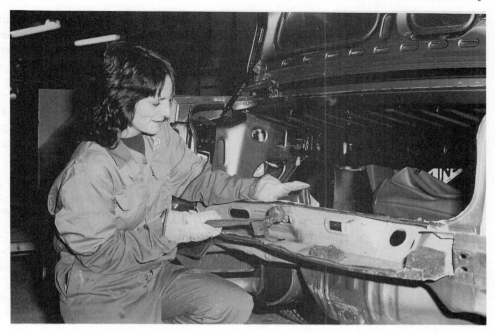

Women still earn, on average, only 60 per cent of what men earn for doing the same job.

- higher levels of divorce, particularly those initiated by the wife and of single parenting with the women as principal parent.

In society at large there have been important developments in the law to give women equal rights in family and employment matters, and protection from sexual discrimination. In spite of these changes, however, women still find themselves disadvantaged in many areas of life, notably those just mentioned. Although laws are in place, their interpretation is loose and the informal systems which operate in the workplace, and in society generally, operate against full equality. For example, women still earn, on average, only 60 per cent of what men earn for doing the same job. In the home, women may now go out to full-time work like their husbands, but they still take primary responsibility for housework. In terms of the role models which we referred to earlier, most children continue to grow up where there is a very clear division between male and female, based on traditional values.

To do

Girls will be girls and boys will be boys. In the socialisation process list ten ways in which girls are brought up to see themselves and behave to be feminine. List another ten ways for boys. Are there any of these which could be changed easily to break the stereotype. Does it matter? You may wish to discuss this in your group.

The fact is that we still bring girls up very differently from boys and from an early age children learn the gender stereotypes and the expected behaviours associated with being male or female. When children watch TV or read the papers these values are reinforced, as they are in the school playground. Since economic and political power tends to be in the control of men these inequalities referred to above are likely to continue. The evidence suggests that women are resistant to taking a more radical role and giving up responsibility for child rearing; therefore they will always be in a minority in the career chase and similarly under-represented in management and discriminating positions in society.

Race

Although only 3 per cent of the British population has an ethnic origin other than British, race relations as a social problem has gained a higher profile than one might assume. There are a number of reasons for this.

- Because of the considerable cultural differences that exist between the indigenous population and those of the main ethnic minorities – Afro-Caribbean, Asian and Chinese – their presence in any community is very noticeable.
- The different ethnic groups arrived within fairly prescribed periods of time: the Afro-Caribbean influx occurred during the early 1950s, the Indian and Pakistani immigrants came in the late 1950s and early 1960s, and the African Asians arrived during the late 1960s. On arrival the majority of immigrants had little money and suffered severe 'cultural shock'; as a result they tended to move to the cheapest housing and areas where their compatriots were already settled. Although the flow of immigrants largely dried up after 1970, as the government clamped down, the pattern of immigrant location has remained largely unchanged and many of the larger cities have neighbourhoods where the majority of residents are from ethnic minority groups.

These concentrations of ethnic groups are, again, highly visible and attract the attention of the media, hence giving an impression of there being a larger population of types of ethnic minorities than there actually is, and from time to time inciting racial prejudice and violence.

- There is still a fairly high level of racial prejudice and discrimination within Britain, and this occasionally results in violent clashes between indigenous whites and ethnic minority groups. In spite of the Race Relations Acts of 1965 and 1976, and the establishment of the Commission for Racial Equality, the level of discrimination in jobs, housing and access to socially valued activities (such as golf clubs) remains high. The police and judiciary are frequently cited as being prejudiced against blacks. The media tend to report on these tensions and create a fear of ethnic minorities, who are then perceived as a threat.

In terms of the socialisation process the major interest will be in how quickly, and to what extent, these different cultural groups become fully assimilated into British society. This, of course, is not a one-way process – for instance, the indigenous whites now have a far more varied diet and enjoy different musical styles such as reggae and rap than was the case 30 years ago – and the host community must itself adapt its ways. However, the evidence is that, while the Afro-Caribbean community is more integrated, Asians are less so. Asian languages and particularly their religions put great barriers in the way of interaction and integration with the indigenous community. Asian family structures are extremely strong and close knit. Asian children are sometimes brought up in strictly controlled environments where communication with whites is restricted to school. Many Asians would like to see Muslim schools which would further divide the communities. However, although all ethnic minority groups include those who are completely opposed to integration, there are a greater number who have moved into the indigenous community and are operating well within it. In order for the situation to improve further there has to be more inter-marriage, greater exposure of the Asian communities, particularly the women, to the indigenous culture and less hostility shown to the ethnic communities by the indigenous population.

People working in the care professions often experience difficult situations with Asian families where the women do not speak English, or their religion forbids them to do something which may be in their best interests. As the traditional family support starts to break down, increasing numbers of Asians will require the support of the state, for care of elders, maternity care, school problems etc. It is important therefore that caregivers are aware of racial and cultural differences, and can take these into consideration when they are carrying out their duties.

To do

Imagine that you are taking an elderly Asian man into care. He is now too frail to be living alone and there is no immediate family. You are to place him in an elderly person's home and you need to make a judgement about which one will best suit his needs. Aside from his health problems, write down a list of factors which you consider will help him to feel, as far as possible, 'at home'.

We have now covered, albeit briefly, the major factors which shape the socialisation process and we will look at the agencies of socialisation in more detail later. It will be clear that the process is extremely complex and that every individual will experience it differently. However, there are important common threads, of roles, of values and attitudes running through the experience and behaviour of everyone who lives in modern British society. There are few sociologists today who would claim, as the American psychologist Watson did, that they could take a dozen infants, selected randomly, and train them to become any kind of specialist : 'doctor, lawyer, artist . . . even beggar man and thief, regardless of his talents, tendencies, abilities, vocation and race of his ancestors'. However, we must always review individual behaviour in the light of a person's upbringing and the nature of the community in which they live.

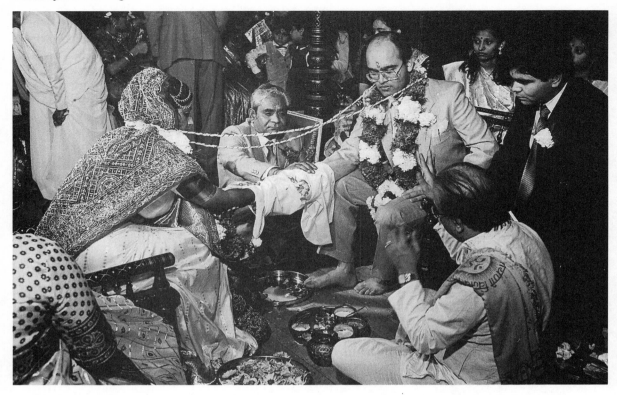

It is important that caregivers are aware of racial and cultural differences, and can take these into consideration when they are carrying out their duties.

The family

In the past the organisation and the culture of societies was a lot simpler than in today's modern Western society. Consequently, the socialisation process was more completely contained within the family, and the cultural material of that society; for instance its religion, or the ways of rearing cattle, were passed down by word of mouth, by demonstration etc. The family was responsible for all its members, whether young or old, and the other agencies that we have referred to were insignificant or non-existent. It is important, therefore, that we look at the family and its role in modern British society before consideration of the influences of other agencies.

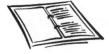

Case study

We have said that the most important period within the socialisation process is childhood, up to and including adolescence, with particular emphasis being placed on the first seven years. This is another reason why the family is central to our concerns in this chapter; at this extremely vulnerable time the infant is totally dependent on its parents and, possibly, other family members. You may have heard of the wolf-child of India, a true story of a boy who was discovered at the age of seven, having apparently been raised by wolves. This boy could not walk or talk, but instead behaved in his human way like the wolves did. He crawled on all fours and made guttural, barking sounds to communicate. He was taken in by missionaries, who attempted to educate him and teach him the basics of human social behaviour. After a year there was some improvement, but much of the behaviour he had learnt could not be erased, and his language in particular would never develop fully because of those crucial missed years.

The institution of the family

What is a family? There is an obvious answer that it is parents, living with their children, under one roof. This describes the most common arrangement in modern, industrial societies, the *nuclear* family. To go further, the nuclear family may have no long-term roots in an area, and although other family members such as parents, brothers and sisters etc. may live nearby, the nuclear family exists independently from them. It is an economic unit, in that one or both parents work to support themselves and their children. Furthermore, the parents may move from area to area for job and financial improvement. The nuclear family is normally small with no more than 2 children (the average is now 1.8), and the relationships between husband and wife, and parents and children, is close and emotionally demanding. The husband and wife will typically share duties around the house, and have similar authority in managing household affairs.

This is an ideal-type family, but in fact there are variations from this theme. The most important are as follows.

- The *extended family* – in the past working-class communities, based around the great industries such as coal and steel, tended to be very stable. The men worked in the factory or down the mine and the women raised the children (of which they were many), looked after the home and often worked part time as well. They were unskilled workers and so there was no reason, or possibility, to move as the boss provided the house and the job. So families grew up together and stayed in the same area. There was much poverty in these communities and no welfare system, apart from that provided by the employer.

  Consequently, the larger family unit was able to provide support at times of illness or other hardship. Today there are still some areas of the UK where the extended family network exists. However, with the decline in traditional heavy and manufacturing industries these communities have been broken up as the need for work forced both parents and children to look for jobs outside the area. Those who were left were often the elderly who couldn't be taken as well. Today, extended families are also found within the Asian communities.

- *Single-parent families* – one of the features of post-war British family life has been the increase in the divorce and in the numbers of single parents who never married. Very often, single-parent families are headed by a woman who may be unable to get a job or adequate child care, and who is therefore on or near the poverty line. The possible consequences of such an increase are discussed below.

- *Reconstructed nuclear families* – with growing rates of divorce and separation, an increasing feature of modern society is the family where partners have either remarried or are simply living together after previously unsuccessful marriages. The effects of such relationships on children is difficult to judge. However, where the parental support is consistent and the separation of parents occurs without too much emotional distress, it is expected that the transition to adulthood should take place satisfactorily.

To do

Find an example, preferably from your own direct experience, of each of the following:

- a nuclear family;
- a nuclear family as part of an extended family;
- a lone-parent family.

Briefly describe each family in terms of:

- how long they have been in the area;
- how long they have been in the dwelling they live in;
- how many children there are;
- whether the mothers work and on what basis – part time, full time etc.;
- the contribution the husband makes to housework as a proportion of the total;
- how many relatives live in the same neighbourhood, then town;
- how often in the last three months the mother had face-to-face contact with her mother;
- who look after the children when the parents go out;
- how many adult friendships are with family members.

Record your views on the differences between the three types of family.

From the results of your investigations different patterns of family life should appear; if they do not this will only reflect the mix of family characteristics that now exist. Many working-class families have now become more affluent – there has been a significant increase in the number of well-paid manual jobs since the Second World War – and may have detached themselves (to differing degrees) from their family roots. Studies have shown how many children from working-class families moved from areas of declining industry to the south for better job prospects during the 1950s and 1960s, and have taken on a very different lifestyle than those they were brought up to. This involves the shift from the extended family patterns to the nuclear family as described above.

The family under attack

There are many public figures, such as politicians and religious leaders, who talk about the collapse of the family, and place the blame for many of our social problems, such as crime and drug taking, at the door of parents. There is certainly an increase in levels of crime and the vast majority of it is committed by young people under the age of 21. At the same time the numbers of people suffering from mental disorders are also on the rise. There is no doubt that the family as an institution is under great pressure, but does that really mean that there is a crisis?

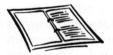

─────── **Case study** ───────

Tracy was 11 when she was accommodated by social services. She and her brother, who was nine at the time, had to be removed from home because of the threat of violence from the parents. Her parents had split up two years previously because of what the courts referred to as 'irreconcilable differences'. The father had been a lorry driver, but had lost his job due to drinking, and then became alcoholic. When drunk he was violent, and beat his wife and the children. The mother also had a drink problem. The family were known to social services, and the mother was receiving support and counselling. However, she was neglecting the children and having great difficulty coping financially or emotionally on her own. The father repeatedly tried to interfere, even after the divorce and a court order restraining him from seeing the family. The children were finally put into long-term foster care with a family near to their home. At this point their father left the area and they did not see him again. The mother fought the care order and was extremely disruptive at the time when the foster family were trying to integrate the children into their family life. She would turn up drunk late at night at the foster home and demand to see the children.

This case study is unfortunately representative of a fairly common occurrence in modern society. In this case alcoholism is a major factor, but it can be substituted for a number of other symptoms of extreme stress or of personal inadequacy, from crime to mental illness. There is a vicious cycle of poverty, deprivation and associated social problems which visit families from generation to generation, and from which each succeeding generation has great difficulty in escaping. However, family breakdown goes much further than the disadvantaged sections of our society. Some of the factors are examined below.

The increase in divorce

The increase in family breakdown can be accounted for in a number of ways.

● The first reason is purely statistical – more people are getting married, people are marrying younger and more divorced couples remarry new partners, so that the overall amount of married years has increased, which in turn means more chances of divorce occurring. However, in real terms, divorce is still on the increase.

- Secondly, the divorce laws have been progressively eased over the 20th century. Not only has this made divorce more of a formality, it has also given women equal access to divorce, and now most divorce suits are initiated by women. One argument in favour of this is that prior to the relaxing of the laws, many families had already broken down, but the wife or husband was trapped by the legal restrictions. In these families the possibility of damage to the children was as great as in the case of parental separation after divorce.

- Thirdly, there has been a significant change in the values and attitudes surrounding marriage. The decline in the influence of the Church and religion has resulted in more permissive sexual behaviour before and during marriage and, it is argued, weakened the strength of commitment to the marriage vows. It does appear that couples take a more businesslike approach to marriage, but there is little evidence to suggest that the ideal of love in marriage or the belief in marriage as a partnership for life have changed as central values. Nevertheless, now that the stigma of being divorced has largely disappeared, couples do not appear to try as hard to keep marriages together in the face of a crisis.

Changing role relationships within the family

Linked to the last point is the change in the relationships between partners. The period since the war has seen women gain far more control over their lives, in the family and, as a closely related issue, in work. Women often have careers and are therefore no longer financially dependent on their partners. The increased access to education and in feminist thinking during the 1960s has transformed the traditional segregation of male/female roles. This has inevitably caused tensions between partners, as men often found the new order difficult to accept. The greater freedom women experience also reflects in women's decisions to file for divorce. It should be pointed out, however, that these changes have probably only affected a minority of women; many are in an unequal relationship, but with all the frustrations of knowing that the situation could be different. In any of these cases there is no conclusive evidence that these different marital roles have an adverse effect on the children.

Social and economic changes

The final factor is the general change in the economy and the behaviour of the workforce. The modern family must be expected to be mobile if the main breadwinner is to improve their position and the family's standard of living. The pace of life is faster; we come into contact with many more people than in the past, but tend to have fewer close friends and less family support. The opportunity for infidelity is much greater, as are the pressures upon marriage caused by the stress of modern living.

What is of interest here is whether the institution of the family is in a state of crisis, and what the consequences of a divorce rate of nearly one in three are. These are certainly critical issues for the welfare state, which relies heavily on the family to provide support for those in need, such as the elderly or the handicapped, and to produce adults who are responsible, contributing members of society. A future society where crime and delinquency are on the increase, where the family elders are neglected and where one-parent families increase the demands on the benefit system is a worrying prospect. With an ageing society and with fewer families in a position to care for themselves, let alone their elders, enormous burdens are likely to be placed on health and social services as they try to support people in their communities.

To do

What do you think about the stability of the family? Using the points raised above, and information gathered from your other reading, list the arguments for and against the view that the family is breaking down. When you have done this try to identify the types of social and economic problems that might a) cause and b) result from family breakdown, together with your reasons why.

Your list of problems raised from the above exercise will probably be quite long, and there is a danger in overstating the potential instability of the family. The bald fact that so many people get divorced hides an important statistic that the majority of divorcees still remarry. Also, there are many instances where families split up in ways which are not full of anger and pain, and which don't damage the children. Many single parents are living happily with their children. The contribution of other factors which influence the development of children, which we have called agencies, such as TV and other media, the peer group of friends and school needs careful attention and we will be investigating these factors below. However, the family unit is of primary importance and must be the centre of your thinking about the socialisation process. There are many more issues to consider than those we have covered here and you are encouraged to read further by reference to the material listed at the back of this book.

The other agencies

To summarise so far, we have looked at the socialisation process in general, how it is defined, how social group, gender and racial origin influence development, and in particular at the influence of the family unit in determining life chances. It may sometimes appear that children who are more disadvantaged have little chance of making a success of their lives. Mrs Thatcher would probably reject that view out of hand, and point to the many successful people who have come from humble or unhappy backgrounds. There is no doubt that there are now different types of provision in society for trying to help people, especially children, to break out of the cycle of deprivation referred to earlier. Much of that effort is focused on the educational system.

The school

Everyone has memories of school days – some good and some bad – but to what extent does the experience shape people's futures? A child who goes to boarding school from an early age is likely to be greatly influenced (as well as by their peer group), but for most children school is a secondary part of their lives. There are two main functions of the educational system in society:

- to ensure that the country has a suitably educated and trained workforce to meet the needs of the economy;
- to pass on from one generation to the next the established values and customs of society, and so promoting order and stability.

In modern society, the family is quite unable to provide the first function itself, but in the case of the second there is more debate. Schools promote the dominant values of society, and if we believe that class is a factor in the organisation of society, then we will see those values as basically middle-class values. Many sociologists have argued that the organisation of schools is a reflection of society at large – the children who work hard and support school values are in the top streams and those who are anti-school are in the bottom streams. This, of course, may not be related to social groups, but other evidence suggests that it is.

To do

A primary school headmistress was quoted in the *Sun* newspaper as saying: 'Many children are already failures at the age of five . . . many of our children are born to fail'. She was referring to the family background, rather than to a child's innate intelligence. What factors in family background would that headmistress be referring to? Provide a list of these factors.

The under-achievement in the educational system of children from working-class backgrounds is a controversial area of discussion. On the one hand there is an implication that some parents are not skilful enough, don't support their children enough or haven't the money to provide some of the things, like extra books, funding for trips etc. that parents are now expected to provide; on the other there are those who criticise schools and teachers who come from and represent middle-class culture and values, and who in a variety of ways, and often unconsciously, discriminate against children from working-class backgrounds. There is powerful evidence from studies by Basil Bernstein that there are clear differences in the language used in schools and that which is used outside, in the family and neighbourhood. Berstein argues that middle-class children are brought up to be familiar with both codes, as he calls them, whereas children from working-class backgrounds only have access to the one (the family and neighbourhood code). Therefore, working-class children are immediately disadvantaged in understanding or relating to what their teachers and books are saying.

The school is a very important feature of the socialisation process. While it can be said that many children are able to improve their life chances compared to their parent's generation through educational success, the fact remains that some 30 per cent of young people leave school at 16 either not properly qualified or having had a negative experience of education. Schools cannot be held responsible for all the problems that are associated with young people – crime, drug taking etc. – but the attitude persists that they are still perpetuating inequalities in opportunity rather than reducing them.

The mass media

The mass media refers to the various systems of communication by which messages, whether they be informative, entertainment or opinion, are transmitted to a mass audience. The main types of mass media are broadcasting – TV and radio – and the press. During the 20th century the importance of the mass media as a part of the socialisation process has grown tremendously.

The difficulty is that we do not have any satisfactory evidence to demonstrate how much influence the media have compared to the other agents. Certainly there is little evidence to show that the mass media actually change people's attitudes. People are selective in what they read as a newspaper and what they watch on TV, and tend to choose programmes which reinforce their own attitudes.

This is true of adults but what about children who are more impressionable and cannot easily separate good from bad in their reading or viewing? When

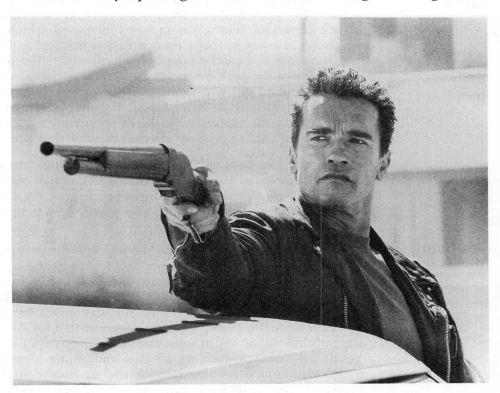

The Terminator – can the media create heroes?

95 per cent of the population have at least one, and frequently more, televisions in their homes, and the average viewing time for some age groups of children has increased to over 21 hours per week, television at least should be seen as an important influence.

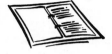

Case study

The Mary Bell case in the 1960s was famous for being one of the first reported examples of the possible dangerous effects of TV. Mary was eight years old when she admitted murdering a three-year-old boy who she was supposed to be looking after. Mary lived in the Gorbals area of Glasgow, in a run-down tenement, and she had taken the little boy to a derelict building and strangled him. What was so shocking was that she said she had seen someone being strangled in a certain way on an episode of The Saint, a popular TV series at the time, and she wanted to try it out herself. After this story broke in the press many commentators were critical of television and the terrible effect they said it had on young children.

Many studies have been carried out to try and establish whether or not television has a lasting effect on children. There is little evidence that sexually explicit material has an impact, but there is more to link the watching of violent TV programmes with aggression. After films like *A Clockwork Orange* and the TV series *Kung Fu* were first shown in the 1960s and early 1970s, violent behaviour among young males increased, which seems to support the theory. However, the main conclusion reached is that TV, of itself, is not damaging and can be positively worth while. The crucial factor is the personality of the person watching and their circumstances. Mary Bell was a very disturbed girl who came from an extremely emotionally deprived background. As a result, being repeatedly left on her own in the tenement, she attached great importance to the TV as a parent substitute. Children who are disturbed tend to be most affected by what they see.

In summary, the mass media can never be the single cause of disturbed or difficult behaviour. However, evidence is contradictory over the lasting effects of TV on children, and it cannot be categorically stated that children's attitudes and tastes are not shaped by what they watch, hear or read.

The peer group

The final category of socialisation to consider is the peer group, or the group of friends that young people have. This feature of the socialisation process only appears as the child approaches adolescence; before then friendships are more superficial and have little influence on the individual's behaviour or development. The influence of the peer group has been given more attention since the 1960s, when teenagers started for the first time to show signs of challenging and in some cases rejecting parental or dominant values. Youth sub-cultures such as hippies and punks developed, and some sociologists argued that a completely separate youth culture was developing, based on the generation gap, and the growing economic and moral independence of teenagers.

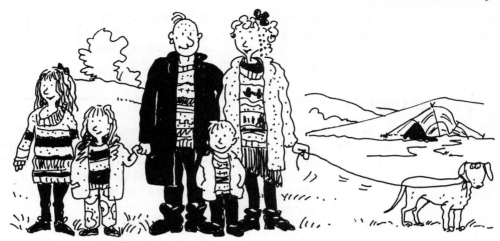

To do

Take one youth sub-culture, and describe the behaviour and beliefs of members of that sub-culture. Explain in what ways they reject traditional, parental values. What other examples are there of these kinds of groups? From your experience how many teenagers are involved in these types of groups – is this a common occurrence?

The evidence suggests that the rejection of parental or traditional values by young people is a temporary phenomenon. It is more about the process of maturing and finding one's own identity as an adult than any collective rejection of society. The numbers of people who continue adopting an alternative lifestyle into adult life are few. The 1960s and 1970s were unusual decades in that they gave birth to such a large number of youth movements. The 'Woodstock generation' are, however, now a part of history.

The peer group clearly becomes very important for teenagers as they approach maturity in providing them with esteem and positive support. Their likes and dislikes will differ from those of their parents, but the effects of socialisation are by this time well rooted and the period of adolescence is a reflection of the earlier periods of the child's upbringing.

The loss of community

As societies change over the years, so the demands upon those who are responsible for the care of individual alter. Modern society has created new and different demands. The decline in the strength of the family unit and the capacity (or willingness) of families to care for their members will put much greater strains on the statutory and voluntary care providers. One consequence of the decline of the family is the increase in the role of secondary socialisation – the school, the mass media etc. Sociologists have referred to the 'loss of community' to describe the effect of people moving around the country for their work, their greater materialism and the inward-looking nature of the nuclear family unit. While one must not get

69

too romantic about the past, where the communities supported one another out of desperate necessity, the future health of society depends to a large extent on the health of communities as social, supportive organisations and the families within them.

Key points

- An individual's life chances and personal development are determined by a combination of inherited characteristics – intelligence, personality etc. – and the social and economic conditions in which they develop.
- The sociological view of personal development is concerned with the interactions between individuals and the social agencies – family, school etc. they are part of.
- The way in which these agencies influence the individual through childhood and adolescence to adulthood is called the socialisation process. There are four main agencies of socialisation in the formative years – the family, the school, the mass media and the peer group.
- The nature of the social interactions within this process are affected by a number of factors, the main ones being social class, gender, race and economic status. These factors clearly influence life chances from the moment a child is born.
- The family is the most important agent of socialisation, but the family has been changing consideraly over the last few decades, and its authority has grown weaker. Increasing family breakdown and social mobility have shifted influence to the other agencies.
- The school is still seen as providing the values and discipline that the society at large wants. There is disagreement, however, about whose society we are talking about, and many sociologists argue that the schools represent the values and behaviour of only a proportion of society – the middle and upper classes.
- The mass media have increased in influence the most, although there is no clear evidence as to how much. Most concern focuses on the influence of TV upon children, in the portrayal of sex and violence, and the way it may be altering the use of leisure time.
- Many sociologists are concerned about the breakdown, not just of families, but of the wider community. The greater mobility of the population, changing work patterns and the growing freedom of children as teenagers have all contributed to what is called 'the loss of community'.

5 *Welfare and society*

In this chapter we will consider the history of the provision of social services in the UK, the type and incidence of problems which are particularly prevalent in society today and the different cash benefits provided by the department of social security for those living close to or below the poverty line. Finally, there will be an attempt to identify whether or not there is a changing pattern of welfare provision being offered in the UK today.

Much of the legislation passed since 1940 forms the basis of the present pattern of the social services or welfare system. The Beveridge Report in 1942, although it has been criticised since, laid the basis for much of the system as it is recognised today.

The Beveridge Report

Sir William Beveridge (later Lord Beveridge) was appointed by the government to review the existing national insurance arrangements. He had had a lifetime's interest in welfare matters and although the government wanted to pass legislation that would 'tidy up' the existing national insurance provisions, he wanted 'a revolution' rather than trying to patch up the system. The report listed five problems confronting a government trying to reconstruct services after the Second World War, and these were disease, squalor, idleness, want and ignorance.

The government accepted most of the recommendations from the report because, at the time, its ideas caught the imagination of the general public who were trying to recover from the after-effects of the Second World War, but it can hardly be referred to as revolutionary because it built largely on existing arrangements and people did not end up with much more money in their pockets because the levels of benefit remained much the same. Beveridge is important, however, because:

- most of the legislation passed after 1940 flowed from this report and formed the basis for our present welfare state;
- the report formed the basis of the present social security system;
- the report abolished the Poor Law and for the first time provided a national minimum of support for everybody;
- for the first time it provided a 'national' system of welfare support rather than a hotch-potch of difference schemes.

In order to understand the developments a little more clearly it is essential to look at other areas of welfare provision, the legislation that was passed in the 1940s and the impact that the Second World War had had on the nation.

Health services

From the beginning of the 20th century there was increasing access to health services for the general public at large, but the Beveridge Report showed the first recognition of the need for a national system of health services because there were many people who were not covered by the national health insurance scheme which was currently in existence. There was a general election in 1945 and Aneurin Bevan, the new Labour health minister, published the National Health Service Bill in 1946, after which the National Health Service as we know it came into being in 1948. It initially provided free health services to everybody, treating physical and mental disorders, and also offering some preventive services.

To do

Using your college or local library find out what were the main provisions of the 1946 National Health Service Bill.

Personal social services

When war broke out in 1939 there was still no universal social work provision as we recognise it today. During the Second World War, when London and many of Britain's large cities were bombed, children were evacuated into the country to live with families they did not know. Families were split apart and it became obvious that there were considerable inequalities between the provision of medical services in the town and country. Many people from the cities were poor, ill-educated and unable to cope.

After the war the government was able to plan and make better social provision for the people of the UK, and in 1948 services were set up nationwide for particular groups of people, including deprived children (the Children's Department), elderly people, physically disabled people and mentally disordered people.

To do

Contact your local social services office and find out how the social services department is organised in your county/city/metropolitan borough. They should be able to provide you with leaflets and an organisation chart. In particular, identify the client groups they are able to help.

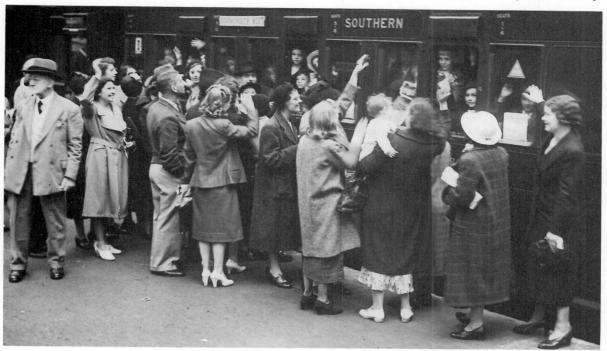

The evacuation of children to the country during the Second World War highlighted the inequalities in caring provision between town and country.

Housing

During the Second World War many homes were either destroyed or seriously damaged as a result of bombing. In 1945 about one in three houses needed renovation or attention.

Under the Housing Act 1946 housing subsidies were introduced and this placed responsibility on local authorities to build new council homes to let. However, housing costs rose steeply after the war and this cut back building programmes, but in 1949 local authorities were able to provide grants for the renovation and improvement of houses.

Council house building continued steadily into the 1980s until the Conservative government under Margaret Thatcher decided that Britain should become 'a nation of home owners' and people who were existing tenants were allowed to purchase their council homes on mortgages at preferential prices. As a result of this policy much of the existing council house stock in this country was sold and since then very few new council homes to rent have been built. Local councils are restricted by central government as to the amount of money they can use to build new council houses or to renovate and repair existing ones. The government is hoping that housing associations will take over the role of building homes for rent to people who cannot afford to buy their own.

Education

During the first 40 years of the 20th century people were beginning to talk about secondary education being available to all children. For the first time the Education Act 1944 or Butler Act (named after RA Butler the minister of state for education) meant that free, full-time education was available to all children up to 15 years of age (later extended to 16), with some opportunities in further and higher education.

After the war Winston Churchill believed that more people should be able to share in the provision of education, and that it should be provided for all and not just a privileged minority. Beveridge, in his report, had also stated that ignorance had to be conquered if the general standard of welfare was to be raised. Again, young men signing up to join the armed forces during the war had highlighted how badly educated some people were and it was obvious that something had to be done about the situation. So the Education Act 1944 provided universal secondary education for all children.

A pattern of change

So, during the 1940s, in the aftermath of the Second World War, changes in legislation in the personal social services, in health, in education, in social security and in housing set the stage for the welfare state as we recognise it today: a system which was to look after everyone 'from the cradle to the

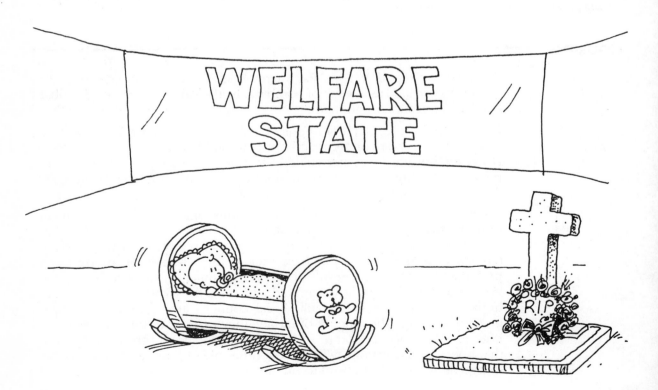

grave' – in other words a welfare system that would look after all of us when we were hard up, when we were sick or when we were faced with personal problems we could not cope with. However, does the present welfare system, just over 40 years on, really look after us 'from the cradle to the grave' and is it realistic to assume that it should? This is a question which will be considered again later in this chapter.

Social problems

To do

As a whole group identify the major social and health problems which face us in society today. In pairs or small groups place them in order of priority and give brief reasons why you put them in that order.

Many of the problems that you will have on your list will include young adults, children, families, old people, disabled people, sick people and mentally ill people who are vulnerable client/patient groups within our society. Not all, but many, of these people will be living either on or below the poverty line, be dependent on state benefits such as pensions and income support, and not be able to afford an adequate diet or always to able to pay their gas and electricity bills, and certainly not able to afford many of life's luxuries.

You probably found it very difficult to put your list of social problems into priority order because everybody has different views, opinions and prejudices. For example, some people will have put the homeless at the top of their list because they feel that a roof over one's head is a basic human right and should therefore be given priority in the pecking order, whereas others consider that Aids sufferers deserve more help because it is a disease which causes intolerable suffering to the patient and their family, and medical science does not yet have a cure.

Let's consider in a little more depth some of the problems which confront our society today and the client/patient groups that are affected by them.

Homelessness You only have to visit cities like London, Birmingham, Newcastle, Belfast or Glasgow to realise that for many people the streets of these cities are home. There are greater numbers of homeless people living on our streets than ever before and not enough shelters or hostels available to provide them with help (that is, those people who want to be helped – for some, living on the streets is a way of life which some people are used to and they don't want it any other way).

These figures have increased for many reasons, but a large contributory factor has been the government's policy on community care. During the

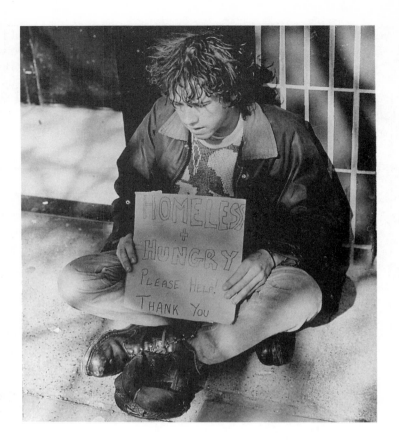

1980s many of the large Victorian mental hospitals have been closed down in the belief that ex-patients would be better off living in smaller hostels, bed and breakfast hotels or half-way hostels in the community. However, there is a problem with this. While some local authorities have successfully rehabilitated mentally ill people, many ex-psychiatric patients have not been so lucky. They have either been in bed and breakfast accommodation, with a lack of community support, or they have been thrown out on to the streets because they have nowhere else to go. Mentally ill people are a very vulnerable group within society.

The policy of the National Health Service has also been to cut back on the numbers of long-stay mental health beds and many people who perhaps need treatment in hospital cannot always get it. They often have to rely on the support of community services, from people like community psychiatric nurses, and if you are homeless then it is unlikely that you are going to find it very easy to have regular contact. For example, a schizophrenic patient may need regular injections in order to keep their symptoms under control and if they are homeless as well their problems are compounded because without a permanent address you can't meet people like the community psychiatric nurse on a regular basis.

To do

Find out what services are provided by the National Health Service and social services in your area for mentally ill people.

Homelessness is also affecting other groups of people in society, including single people and families. Many families are currently living in bed and breakfast accommodation because they have no permanent home and this situation is not likely to get any better because government policy on housing over the 1980s has encouraged people to try and buy homes of their own. In 1989 about 65 per cent of the population owned their own homes. Some people took on large mortgages which they couldn't really afford, then perhaps lost their jobs and eventually got into arrears with their payments and lost their homes. As Table 5.1 shows, between 1981 and 1990 statutory homelessness (homeless people which the local authority accepted responsibility for rehousing) as a result of a court order following mortgage default or rent arrears multiplied by 2.5 times.

Table 5.1 Homeless households found accommodation by local authorities: by reason for homelessness, 1981 and 1991

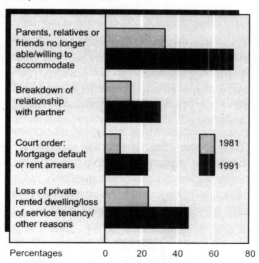

Source: *Social Trends 23* (HMSO, 1993)

As we saw in Chapter 4, the government, over the 1980s, also allowed local authorities to sell many of their council houses to existing tenants, while restricting the amount of money to be spent on building new homes for people with affordable rents. While it is obviously a good idea for as many people as possible to own their own homes, it has also meant that many single parents, young people and families find themselves often on never-ending council waiting lists and in the mean time live in temporary, unsatisfactory accommodation.

To do

Imagine you are a single parent living in bed and breakfast accommodation with Sean aged two years and Matthew who is six months old. You have to cook breakfast on a small stove and do everything in this one room. Putting yourself in her place, describe a typical day. Try to imagine what your feelings would be like.

Young people have also been affected. They come to large cities looking for employment, or have to leave their families for various reasons, perhaps cannot find work and end up without a roof over their heads. It is also difficult for young people to find private rented accommodation at an affordable price and not many local authorities can offer rented accommodation for single young people.

To do

Contact your local district/town/city council housing department and find out how many people are on their waiting list for housing. What sort of provision do they make for families who are homeless?

**Unemploy-
ment**

Unemployment is at a very high level in the early 1990s and the figures for the number of people who are unemployed are still rising (early 1993). Table 5.2 shows that the numbers of people unemployed dropped steadily between 1986 and 1989, but rose to the 2.5 million point in the early months of 1991. In early 1993 the numbers of unemployed people are around 3 million.

This means that many are not only finding it increasingly difficult to find further employment, but they are also reliant on state benefits like

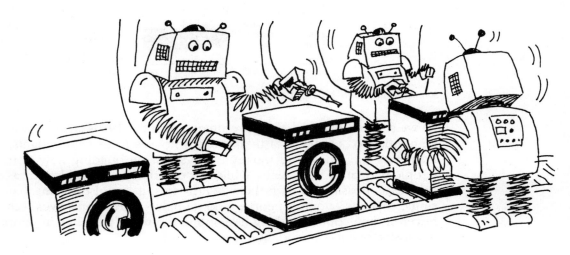

Table 5.2 Unemployment and vacancies

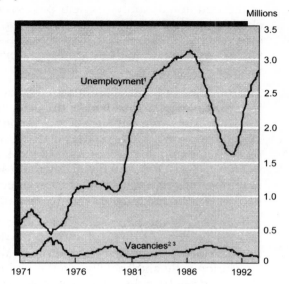

1 Seasonally adjusted unemployment (claimants aged 18 and over).
2 About one-third of all vacancies are notified to job centres.
3 Vacancy data prior to 1980 are not consistent with current coverage.

Source: *Social Trends 23* (HMSO, 1993)

unemployment benefit and income support, which in turn means that families suffer because they are unable to maintain the same standard of living as they could when the breadwinners were in employment.

There are many reasons why unemployment has been on the increase in the early 1990s. Historically, over the last 20 or 30 years, much of the UK's traditional industry base has changed. For example, industries like steel making, ship building, coal mining and the car industry have declined. These were labour-intensive industries and, even where industry has survived, technology has meant that fewer people are employed to do the same job. For example, robots in the car industry now carry out jobs which people used to do. People now have to be prepared to retrain and develop new skills in order to undertake different jobs. Fifty years ago a person may have trained for one job for life, whereas now people have to be prepared to retrain and perhaps undertake two or three different jobs in their working lives.

The problem of unemployment is also linked closely to education and training, and young people are also finding it increasingly difficult to stay in work. In 1993, the trade barriers in the European Community were lifted and theoretically anyone from another EC country can come and seek employment in the UK and vice versa. In order to compete effectively in such a competitive climate it seems likely that the government will have to develop improved training programmes for all.

The changing pattern of family life

As we saw in Chapter 4 the family unit is taking on a new shape. Instead of the traditional family (nuclear pattern) of mother, father and one or two children, many children are now growing up in single-parent and step-parent families. In fact, if divorce statistics continue to rise more children will be growing up in these kinds of families by the end of the 20th century than will grow up in nuclear families.

The number of single-parent families has steadily increased over the last few years, and this has had both social and economic implications. Many single parents are dependent on income support, either because their children are too young and they can't work or there is inadequate child-care provision, or single parents want to work but they cannot because they are unable to find a job which will pay them sufficient money to be able to live, pay their bills and afford child care when they cannot be there to provide it. This is sometimes called the poverty trap.

In many cases, the parent who ends up caring for the children after divorce takes a drop in income. They may be dependent on income support or maintenance from the ex-partner and this reflects economically, psychologically and socially, on the children in the family. For example, a child may not be able to have outings and treats which other school friends are able to enjoy and this can be very upsetting to a child and the parent who cannot afford them. Emotionally, the children may be missing the partner who has left the family home as well. Although divorce can be a very upsetting experience for a child, they are usually resilient and can recover from it.

As a result of the increased divorce rate many children now live in step-parent families when their mother or father remarries.

To do

Find out what types of family the members of your group belong to. Draw a pie chart to illustrate your results. You may want to include other types of families, for example families where the children are adopted, or foster families.

Rising crime statistics

It is a fact that the UK is currently faced with rising crime statistics and that young people are often involved. As you can see in Table 5.3 the crime rate in England and Wales continued to rise steadily during the 1980s, and shows no sign of abating. It is not only minor crimes which are on the increase. Society is becoming more violent and more serious crimes like rape are on the increase.

The media make us aware of new kinds of crime which young people are becoming involved in, and the kinds of things which are on the increase include young people taking and driving away cars, and so-called joyriding. It is worth stressing that the young people involved in these types of criminal activity are in the minority and, of course, television and the newspapers

Table 5.3 Notifiable offences recorded by the police: by type of offence

Thousands

	England & Wales			Scotland			Northern Ireland		
	1971	1990	1991	1971	1990	1991	1971	1990	1991
Notifiable offences recorded									
Violence against the person	47.0	184.7	190.3	5.0	13.6	15.5	1.4	3.4	4.0
Sexual offences , of which,	23.6	29.0	29.4	2.6	3.2	3.1	0.2	0.8	0.9
rape and attempted rape	0.8	3.4	4.0	0.2	0.5	0.5	..	0.1	0.1
Burglary	451.5	1,006.8	1,219.5	59.2	101.7	116.1	10.6	14.8	16.6
Robbery	7.5	36.2	45.3	2.3	4.7	6.2	0.6	1.6	1.8
Drugs trafficking	..	10.0	11.4	..	2.8	3.3	..	-	-
Theft and handling stolen goods	1,003.6	2,374.4	2,761.1	104.6	255.2	284.3	8.6	29.3	32.0
of which, theft of vehicles	167.6	494.2	581.9	17.1	36.1	44.3	..	7.0	8.4
Fraud and forgery	99.8	147.9	174.7	9.4	25.0	26.4	1.5	4.2	4.8
Criminal damage	27.0	733.4	821.1	22.0	86.4	89.7	7.4	2.2	2.4
Other notifiable offences	5.6	21.1	23.2	5.9	43.2	48.1	0.5	1.0	1.0
Total notifiable offences	1,665.7	4,543.6	5,276.2	211.0	535.8	592.8	30.8	57.2	63.5

Source: *Social Trends 23* (HMSO, 1993)

don't tend to publicise the good work that many young people do for all kinds of groups of disadvantaged people in the community.

Drugs, alcohol, smoking and solvent abuse

Substance abuses particularly affect young people, and can easily ruin and upset lives if they get out of hand. It is a depressing fact that most of these addictions are on the increase.

Smoking is perhaps considered by some to be the least serious of any of these addictions, but it worries many health promoters that large numbers of young people start smoking at a very early age. Many young people start smoking by the age of 11, and the problem is how to make them realise that smoking at that age can seriously damage their health in later years, making them particularly vulnerable to different kinds of cancers and heart disease. The sale of cigarettes to young people under the age of 16 years is banned by statute.

Alcohol, drugs and solvent abuse are also on the increase. Table 5.4 uses data extracted from surveys of alcohol consumption in England and Wales, as carried out by the Office of Population Censuses and Surveys in 1987, 1988 and 1989. It shows a comparison of alcohol consumption by sex and social class.

Heavy consumption of alcohol can lead young people into problems if their habit gets out of hand. Young people can often become involved in crime when they have been drinking, for example theft, taking and driving away motor vehicles, causing problems at football matches or generally committing vandalism.

Taking drugs intravenously (by injection) makes people more vulnerable to Aids, especially if they share needles. New drugs such as Ecstasy are now

Table 5.4 Alcohol consumption: by sex and social class, 1987 and 1989

England & Wales				Units of alcohol
	Males		Females	
	1987	1989	1987	1989
Professional	11.4	10.2	4.3	5.3
Managerial and				
junior professional	15.4	15.0	6.1	5.3
Other non-manual	14.0	11.8	5.3	3.5
Skilled manual	15.4	13.1	4.6	4.1
Semi-skilled manual	12.5	16.3	3.4	3.2
Unskilled manual	17.3	14.8	3.7	4.1
All persons aged				
16 and over	14.5	13.9	4.8	4.2

Source: *Social Trends 23* (HMSO, 1993)

coming on to the market and young people are encouraged, perhaps at parties, to try them for fun. Drug taking of any kind has serious consequences and when it becomes a habit it can lead people into stealing, lying, prostitution and many other kinds of social problems just in an attempt to be able to afford their addiction.

Increasing numbers of elderly people

There are increasing numbers of elderly people living in the UK and this continues to put pressure on social, health and community services in terms of resources and finance. A government White Paper, entitled *Caring for People – Community care in the next decade and beyond*, notes that the elderly population in the 85+ age bracket is projected to continue rising up to the year 2001, as it is in the 75 to 84 age bracket. Old people, particularly women, in these age groups are living longer because of better standards of living, and improvements in science and medicine. Indeed, 19 per cent of our total population is elderly, and this has serious implications for society.

The likelihood is that at some stage in their lives many old people are likely to need care. Some old people are cared for by their families, but many families, for varied reasons (see Chapter 4), are not able to offer this care and so old people have to become reliant on statutory and private provision.

In recent years there has been a sharp increase in the numbers of private rest homes and nursing homes opening up, which has been a direct result of government policy, not only in encouraging private enterprise, but also in admitting that the statutory services, namely social services and the NHS, cannot cope with the increasing demands for care which an ever-growing elderly population is making on resources. The government may pay something towards maintaining a person in a rest home or nursing home if they do not have adequate financial resources themselves.

It is also important to remember that many older people do not rely on any of these services and are able to live happy, fulfilled lives in retirement. Many older people still go on working part time or they may undertake voluntary work in the community to help other people.

To do

Find out the current rates of state pension for a married couple and a single person. Imagine you are a 78-year-old widow living alone in a two-bedroomed bungalow. You own the property. Draw up a weekly budget for all the things you need to pay for out of your weekly pension, for example, food, gas, electricity bills and so on. How easy do you think it is to manage?

Aids

The HIV virus, which causes Aids, is transmitted sexually, in blood and blood products, and can be passed from a mother who is infected to her unborn child. The number of reported cases is, unfortunately, on the increase.

Table 5.5 shows numbers of Aids cases by the end of March 1991 per million population in EC countries. The EC average was 135 cases per million and Great Britain is well below that with 78 cases per million population. France has the most serious Aids problem in the EC with approximately 257 cases per million population. However, the problem is much more serious in North America, Africa and Asia. It is estimated that Africa has five-sixths of the world's HIV-positive women.

So far more men than women are affected, but it is a fallacy to believe that only homosexuals are affected by Aids. The disease is spreading in the

Table 5.5 Reported Aids cases: EC comparison, 1992

Country	Rate per million population
United Kingdom	
Belgium	
Denmark	
France	
Germany	
Greece	
Irish Republic	
Italy	
Luxembourg	
Netherlands	
Portugal	
Spain	
EUR 12	

Rate per million population: 0 60 120 180 240 300 360

Source: *Social Trends 23* (HMSO, 1993)

heterosexual community and sexual intercourse between heterosexuals is now the main route of transmission. Intravenous drug users are particularly at risk, especially if they share needles which could be infected.

There is much prejudice against people who have Aids or who are HIV positive and although medical science is making rapid advances, there is, as yet, no cure for Aids. Therefore, the main weapon in the fight against it is good health education for everybody; particularly those people in the population who are identified as running a high risk of being infected. The government has funded various health education programmes, including television advertising campaigns.

People who may have been exposed to the virus should not be encouraged to donate blood, organs or semen, and should be encouraged to modify their sexual behaviour to avoid practices that are particularly likely to transmit the virus. On a note of reassurance, the screening of potential blood donors for antibodies to HIV and the heat treatment of blood products has virtually eliminated the risk to recipients of blood in the UK.

Ethnic minorities

As Table 5.6 shows, the UK is a multi-cultural society. Families from India, Pakistan, Africa and Asia have made the UK their home. Many ethnic minority children have been born here and may never have lived in their parents' native country. This means that people with many different lifestyles and different religions are now living side by side.

In recent years violent outbreaks have occurred in the UK (for example, Toxteth in Liverpool and Brixton in London) because different ethnic groups have found it impossible to live side by side. Some Anglo-Saxon whites are prejudiced against certain ethnic groups, feeling that they have no right as

Table 5.6 Households with dependent children: by ethnic group of head, 1989 and 1991 average

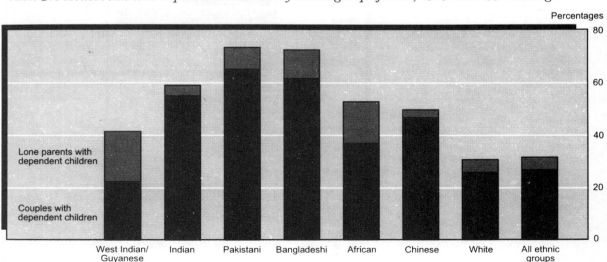

Source: *Social Trends 23* (HMSO, 1993)

immigrants to live in the UK, and benefit from 'their' education, social and health care services, and take 'their' jobs. Surely this is a very narrow view to take.

It is vital to remember that many families who were once immigrant families have had children who have grown up here and who are now marrying and raising families of their own. In other words, they are second-generation families who rightly regard the UK as their home. Many of these families originate from India and Pakistan. The reason for this is that there was a lot of fighting and unrest in India in 1947 after the fall of the Raj, when India was divided up to form the countries of India and Pakistan. Many families emigrated after that, seeking a better life for themselves.

A potential source of immigrants may be from among the Chinese population of Hong Kong who hold UK passports. Some of these people want to leave the British colony and settle in the UK or in other Commonwealth countries, before Hong Kong is handed over to the Chinese authorities in 1997. The Hong Kong people fear that if they stay in the colony the Chinese authorities may not allow them to leave, and they may stop the development of business and commerce for which Hong Kong is renowned. Many people emigrate because of a fear of political repression in their own countries.

To do

In small groups discuss what particular problems ethnic minority groups might have in integrating into existing welfare/health programmes.

When considering the changing patterns of social and health problems in society, it is important to remember that many of these problems overlap and cannot be considered in isolation. For example, a single parent who is on income support may have a drug problem; or a young person who is unemployed and receiving unemployed benefit may not have a stable home life, and may already have a criminal record; or an old person may be living in poor housing conditions, and below the poverty line. The other thing to remember is that many people in society live happy, well-adjusted lives and do not necessarily experience any or all of these kinds of problems which have been mentioned. It is very easy when you start to consider society's problems to begin to see a distorted picture.

The welfare benefits system

Many of the people who experience the kinds of problems we have been considering will be claiming benefit and living on or below the poverty line, but it is important to ask what *is* the poverty line?

The poverty line

The poverty line is really an imaginary line which is set by the government. Many changes were made by the government to the social security system in 1988 and prior to this people who today are on income support were known as supplementary benefits claimants. Each year the government sets scales of allowances for people on income support. These allowances bear no relation to the wages of people in work and if people fall below these levels of income they are considered to be below the poverty line.

The concept of 'relative poverty' is also used to judge who is poor in society today. People are considered poor if they cannot maintain the lifestyle of an 'average' person or family in society. For example, people on income support may find it difficult, through lack of money, to provide their family with an adequate diet which includes fresh meat and vegetables every day, or to furnish their home with the most basic of items such as a cooker, refrigerator and television, or they may not be able to afford their heating bills.

Evidence suggests that poverty has not lessened. A television survey called 'Breadline Britain' indicated that there are probably some 10 million people living on or below the poverty line in Britain in the early 1990s. Some of the reasons for this are:

- rising numbers of unemployed people;
- the increasing numbers of elderly people drawing retirement pensions;
- the increasing numbers of one-parent families;
- inflation – the increasing rise in the cost of living;
- people retiring at an early age;
- people being made redundant.

Types of benefit

There are three main types of benefit:

- contributory benefits;
- non-contributory benefits;
- means-tested benefits.

Contributory benefits

People are entitled to receive contributory benefits based on the amount of national insurance contributions they have paid. National insurance contributions are based on a percentage of total income, which people who are working pay every week. This money then goes towards paying for various benefits and towards financing the National Health Service. The main contributory benefits are:

- unemployment benefit;
- statutory sick pay;
- invalidity benefit;
- old age pension;
- maternity benefits;
- widow's benefits.

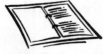

Case study

Mr Sahni came to England from Uganda with his wife and two children about ten years ago. Shushila is 11, Hari is 14 and they attend local schools. They settled in an area of Southampton and Mr Sahni worked as a plant operative in a large factory producing vans. Mrs Sahni stayed at home to look after the family. About ten weeks ago Mr Sahni was made redundant from his job, and has had to sign on and claim unemployment benefit. Find out how much unemployment benefit a married man with two children, and whose wife is not working, would be entitled to claim on a weekly basis.

Non-contributory benefits

These benefits are paid without people making contributions from their weekly income. The main ones are:

- attendance allowance;
- mobility allowance;
- child benefit;
- invalid care allowance;
- severe disablement allowance;
- disablement allowance.

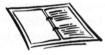

Case study

Miss Harris cannot work because she stays at home to care for her elderly mother who suffers from multiple sclerosis. Her mother, Edna, aged 67 is a wheelchair user and needs help from her daughter in order to go to the toilet, and with washing and bathing, although the district nurse is able to offer some help with this. Miss Harris sometimes has disturbed and sleepless nights, because she has to get up and turn her mother over in bed, as she is now not able to do this for herself. She also has to help her on to the commode at night. Which of the above benefits would Miss Harris and her mother Edna be able to claim? Find out how much they would receive between them per week.

Means-tested benefits

You are entitled to means-tested benefits without paying national insurance contributions. However, the amount of benefit you receive may be reduced by any income which you are receiving or amounts of savings which you have. The main ones are:

- income support;
- family credit;
- social fund.

Income support

This is a weekly allowance for people whose financial resources fall below the basic amount set by the government (poverty line). There are certain weekly amounts of income support laid down for an adult, a couple and children.

People on income support are also entitled to other non-cash benefits, for example free prescriptions, fares paid for certain hospital visits, free eye tests, dental treatment and so on.

Social fund

The social fund provides for one-off payments to people who need a lump sum of money. For example, if someone is on income support and they move house they might need money to buy a new cooker, beds for the children or floor coverings. Such a request is normally met from the social fund in the form of a loan which has to be repaid out of that person's weekly allowance. This is not very easy to do if you are living on income support.

The social fund has been criticised frequently, because many people do not get a loan when they request it. This is because each social security office is allocated so much money per year and once this money has been paid to claimants there is no more money available until the next financial year.

Family credit

This benefit is payable as a top-up to weekly income where families are living on a particularly low wage. One parent must be working for at least 24 hours a week in order to claim family credit.

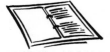

Case study

Yvonne Barrett is a single, black parent with three children. Her parents emigrated to the UK from Trinidad in the 1950s, so Yvonne has grown up here. Her children are Sasha aged ten, Michaela aged seven and Tom who is three. The family live in a rented, seventh-floor council flat.

Yvonne would like to go back to work. She used to work as an insurance clerk, but unfortunately she cannot find a job which will pay enough to enable her to go back to work, so she is dependent on income support. Find out how much she is entitled to each week on income support. What other benefits can she claim as a single parent on income support?

Housing benefit

This scheme provides payments for people who cannot afford to pay their rent, council tax or mortgage. For example, a person who is on income support is automatically entitled to housing benefit and people who are dependent on income support will not have to pay the government's new council tax whereas with the community charge they were responsible for paying 20 per cent of the full amount.

Other people, even if they are working and on a low income, are entitled to receive some help, but the amount varies according to family size, income and the amount of savings a family has.

A changing pattern of welfare?

It is evident that poverty over the last 20 years has not decreased. Indeed, several factors have added to the numbers of people who are dependent on state benefits. These are:

- a larger elderly population, who are living longer;
- a rising number of unemployed people;
- an increasing number of people who are losing their homes because of mortgage arrears and repossession of homes;
- rises and peaks in the cost of living – inflation;

- an ever-increasing divorce rate with the UK having the second highest rate in Europe after Denmark;
- an increasing number of single-parent families.

Increasingly the statutory caring and health services are becoming more dependent on the voluntary and private sectors to supplement the services which they provide. Government policy is actively encouraging an increased reliance on the private and voluntary sectors in terms of providing care packages for a range of client groups. Services for elderly people provides a good example of this. Through the Community Care Act, which became law in April 1993, although social service departments will be the lead body in the structure, they will use voluntary and private agencies in order to put together care packages for their clients/patients. Many voluntary agencies such as Age Concern and Help the Aged provide services which supplement the statutory bodies in providing services for elderly people. Also, there has been a vast increase in the services provided for retired and elderly people by the private sector as a direct result of the government encouraging an open competitive market for welfare services.

Key points

- Changes in legislation in the personal, social services, education, health, housing and social security areas formed the basis for the welfare state as we know it today.
- The Beveridge Report was important in instigating these changes.
- Certain client/patient groups make more demands on statutory, voluntary and private services than others.
- Some ten million people live on or below the poverty line and are dependent on a range of state benefits.
- There are three main types of benefit:
  – contributory benefits;
  – non-contributory benefits;
  – means-tested benefits.
- Problems which face society change as a result of current government social, health and economic policies.
- There is a changing pattern of welfare. Statutory services rely on voluntary and private services to help meet increased demands in providing care packages.
- The government wishes to place more emphasis on care in the community for a range of patient/client groups through the Community Care Act which came into force in April 1993.
- The government has encouraged the expansion of the private care sector, particularly for elderly people.

6 *Communication skills*

For those wishing to pursue a career in the caring professions language, and the ability to use it effectively, is one of the most important tools to acquire. Whether it is verbal, written or non-verbal communication, language allows carers to find out how their clients/patients are feeling, what problems they have to face now and in the future, and what kind of relationship they are building with them as carers. It also allows carers to carry out assessments, together with clients/patients and other members of the team in order to plan for their future.

In order to be an effective communicator it is important to have an understanding of the actual process and what is happening between people when they are communicating – the communication process.

The communication process

To do

Cover up the definition below and jot down what you think the word communication means.

Communication is the ability to impart knowledge or information, or exchange thoughts, feelings or ideas by speech writing, gestures and so on. This sounds very simple and straightforward, but all kinds of difficulties get in the way of effective communication. First we should consider how communication takes place.

Communication models

Model 1

Sender → Message → Receiver

Model 2

Model 3

In the first model communication is a one-way process. You could think of it as leaving a message on a telephone answering machine and getting no response. You leave your message on the tape and no one is able to respond to it. In real life communication is rarely like this.

In the second model the arrows point in both directions, namely to and from both the sender and receiver, indicating that communication is a two-way process. A person thinks of a message that they want to send, chooses the mode and channel of communication which they are going to use to send their message and puts it into the appropriate 'language'. Almost at the same time the other person is receiving the message and interpreting the 'language'. We give feedback to the sender of the message to indicate whether or not we have received and understood the message. We give feedback to the other person by using non-verbal communication, asking questions and by giving continuation messages (paralanguage or intonation and gesture).

In the third model communication becomes a multi-way process. An example of this might be a chairperson at a meeting communicating with several people and each person responding in turn to what is being said.

Modes of communication

We communicate in many different ways, not only by using words. Sometimes these way of communicating are referred to as *modes*. Below is a list of some modes which we use to communicate:

- spoken words;
- written words;

- facial expressions;
- paintings;
- mime;
- mathematical symbols;
- chemical symbols;
- computer language;
- photographs;
- touch and physical contact;
- sign language.

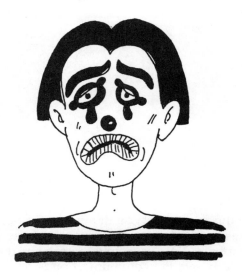

To do

Add as many other modes of communication as you can to this list.

You probably now have quite a long list, with some modes being more difficult to use than others. For example, we all use facial expressions without thinking, but you need to learn how to use a simple, accepted sign language like Makaton. In a sense all modes of communication are codes, but some codes may be more difficult to use than others. For example, you need to be trained in the use of computer language to use it effectively. If we refer back to our communication models, in order for effective communication to take place it is necessary for both the sender and the receiver to understand the mode of communication being used.

If you decide to send a message using sign language and the receiver does not understand sign language then obviously your message will not get across clearly. So both the sender and receiver of the message must be able to understand and interpret the chosen mode of communication.

Sending the message

Having decided on the most appropriate mode for sending your message you need to think about how to get that message across. This is often called the *channel of communication* and refers to the best way of sending your message. Examples of channels of communication are:

- telephones;
- memos;
- letters;
- books;
- face-to-face contact;
- newspapers;
- fax machines.

For example, if you worked as a care assistant in a rest home for elderly people and you were asked to organise an outing for some of the residents you could send them all a memo, but that would be a very formal channel of communication to choose in order to get your message across. It would be much more informal and friendly to go and chat to each person, and ask their opinion about the outing.

When sending a message, in order to communicate effectively, it is necessary to consider the following questions.

- What mode of communication will express you message most effectively?
- What modes are available to you?
- How many receivers do you have to send you message to?
- Who are your receivers, e.g. children, old people, hearing impaired people?
- Where are your receivers, e.g. distance?
- How quickly do you need to send your message?
- What is the approximate cost of sending your message?

Developing your communication skills

In this chapter and Chapter 7 on interpersonal skills the following communication skills will be considered in more depth:

- written;
- non-verbal communication, e.g. body language;
- speaking and listening.

These communication skills will be considered as separate elements, but it is important to remember that in daily life we are often using them all simultaneously.

For example, when you are speaking at a case conference you are bringing many of your communication skills into play. You may have prepared some notes about what you are going to say, you will listen to what other colleagues have to say about a particular client, you may speak and make a contribution yourself and finally your body language, including the way you are dressed and your gestures and facial expression, will be saying something to the other group members about the way you are feeling.

Before considering these skills in more depth it is important to remember that you will also have to communication with clients/patients who will have to communicate with you in their own special way.

Visually impaired clients

Clients who are visually impaired, either totally blind or partially sighted, will use touch as a method of communicating in order to get a 'picture' in their mind of how someone appears as a person. They may use their hands to touch a person's face and hair. Be prepared for this. They may also be more sensitive to subtle changes in people's tone of voice.

Elderly people who have perhaps lost their sight later in life need help with written communication, for example personal letters or guidance in signing cheques.

Hearing impaired clients

If you work with hearing impaired clients you may have to learn a whole new method of communicating!

For example, you may have to learn a sign language like Makaton in order to communicate effectively. However, many hearing impaired people use lip-reading as a means of communication. If you are being lip-read it is important to speak slowly and clearly, and face the hearing impaired person so that they can watch your lips. Beards and moustaches should also be trimmed as necessary.

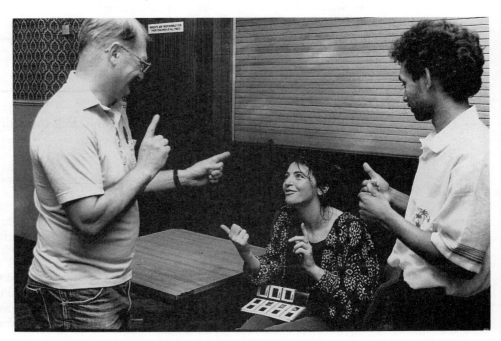

To do Ask a friend to cover their ears firmly, you speak two or three sentences and see if your friend can repeat what you were saying. Reverse roles and try again! How difficult was this?

Other client groups

Other clients may also have difficulty in communicating. For example, a person who is very depressed may not want to talk to you and sometimes just a reassuring hand on the shoulder, without speaking, may make that person feel that you do care and are trying to understand.

Some people with severe learning difficulties, elderly or young, may have a very limited vocabulary, and there may be instances when you have to speak on a client's behalf, for example at a review or case conference. This is a big responsibility.

To do As a group discuss what other situations you can think of where there might be a problem in communicating with clients/patients. Identify what these problems are.

Written skills

Letter writing

There are two kinds of letters that carers may be called upon to write. They are:

- personal letters for clients who may be unable to do this for themselves;
- business letters on behalf of a client or for the organisation which employs you.

To do Jot down how you begin and end a letter when you know the person you are writing to and how you begin and end a letter when you just have the name of the organisation.

Here are some pointers to remember when writing business letters.

- If it is a complicated letter make some rough notes first.
- Always keep in mind the person(s) to whom you are writing, for example are they young or old, male or female?
- Use clear and precise language that you know the recipient will understand.
- Use a heading after 'Dear Sir/Madam' to summarise the contents of your letter.
- Avoid the use of jargon which the recipient may not understand.

- Use an appropriate tone.
- Use appropriate conventions of paragraphing, spelling and grammar. It does matter! If you can't spell very well keep a pocket dictionary in your desk drawer!
- Develop your letter logically. Refer to any correspondence and state why you are writing in your opening paragraph.
- Always remember that a business letter written by you represents the organisation you work for.
- Letter writing is FUN!

Memos

Memos are internal forms of communication within an organisation written between colleagues and departments with copies going to other people for information only. They can be about a range of topics concerning decisions made within organisations. For example a memo might request you to attend a case conference on a certain day or it might ask you to make some observations about how well a new elderly client is settling into the residential home that you work for and to make a short written report or contribute towards an assessment on that elderly person.

Most organisations have pre-printed forms for memos. They can be handwritten or typed as they are a less formal means of communication than a business letter which is being sent outside the organisation.

Here are some pointers to remember when writing memos.

- You know who you are writing to so you can get on with your message without the opening paragraph you would use in a business letter.
- Refer to any relevant memos or previous conversations if necessary.
- Keep your message brief and to the point.
- Keep your use of jargon to a minimum. Some is all right since you and the recipient share the same business, i.e. caring.
- No formal opening or closing as in a letter is necessary.
- Just initial or sign your message at the end.
- A memo is a less formal piece of communication than a letter.
- Always ask yourself if a memo is the best way to get your message across. For example, if you don't need a written record an internal telephone call may be quicker.

To do

On pages 99–101 are three examples of letters and one memo written by or to people working in the caring field. In small groups analyse them and consider the following points.

- Is the language and meaning clear?
- Is the tone of the letter appropriate?
- Is the layout accurate and correct?

Now choose one of the letters and write a reply to it.

Letter 1

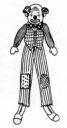

Funtime Summer Play Project
19 Smithies Crescent
Oxford
OX1 3TH
Tel: (0865) 781456

Organiser: Janet Burrows

19 May 1993

Tutor in Charge
Community Care Department
Oxford College of Further Education
Oxenall Road
OXFORD   OX3 4BH

Dear Sir

<u>PLAY PROJECT 27 JULY 1993 – 27 AUGUST 1993</u>

We will be running our play project again this year for
children aged four to nine years whose mothers are working
during the school summer holidays or where a child may have
been referred to us by the social services department for a
variety of reasons.

We are looking for three young people who may be able to
assist us for this period with the day-to-day care of the
children. They should be confident about caring for a group
of three to four children, organising appropriate
activities for them and be available to travel to and from
the children's homes night and morning on the mini-bus
transport which we will be providing.

We will be able to pay approximately £1.50 per hour. Can
you please let us know whether any of your students are
interested. If you have any other queries please contact me
on the above number.

Yours faithfully

Janet Burrows.

JANET BURROWS
PROJECT ORGANISER

Letter 2

19 Leander Road
Worksop
Notts
NG13 5HT
Tel: (0909) 457132

26 September 1993

Social Services Department
12 The Quadrant
Stevenage
Herts SG8 9BB

Dear Sir

Re: Maud Carruthers

My mother is 83 years old, living alone in a two-bedroom bungalow and I am extremely worried about her. I live a long way away, have a family of my own and I am also a single parent and this makes it very difficult for me to visit my mother.

Recently I have had several telephone calls from my mother's neighbour, Mrs Geddes, saying that on at least two occasions she has found my mother wandering in the street not knowing where she was going. She didn't seem to remember where she lived either. Mrs Geddes very kindly took her home, made her a cup of tea and made sure that she was all right.

I am very worried because I can't come and see my mother and she is not on the telephone so please can someone visit her as soon as possible? I really am very worried.

Yours faithfully

Linda Johns

Letter 3

Sheredees Health Centre
Upton Way, Stevenage   SG12 9EB
Tel: (0438) 976012

Dr Penny Bryant, MB, DRCOG
Dr Jim McCullen, MB
Dr Geoffrey Boult, MB

The Social Services Department,
12 The Quadrant,
STEVENAGE   SG8 9BB

13 September 1993

Dear Sirs,

RE: SALLY HEDGES (DOB 12.3.40)

The above 53-year-old lady who suffers from multiple
sclerosis, and has done so for the past ten years, lives
with her husband and two teenage children in a
three-bedroom semi-detached house at 33 Cedar Close,
Stevenage.

She has recently become depressed and now uses, almost
permanently, a wheelchair. Her husband who goes out to
work has always cared for her but he is finding it
increasingly difficult to do so. In particular, since she
has been depressed he worries about leaving her alone all
day.

At present our district nursing service goes in daily to
get Mrs Hedges up and a nursing assistant goes in once a
week to bath Mrs Hedges. However, I feel she needs more
support than we can offer and would be grateful for your
assessment of this patient.

Yours faithfully,

Penny Bryant

PENNY BRYANT

The following is an example of a memo.

MEMO

TO: Ms Jane Barrett
Care Assistant

FROM: Colin Wilkinson
Assistant Officer
in Charge

DATE: 20 August 1993

Copies: Ms Janet Parker
Mr Len Sutton

SUBJECT: LEONIE GREEN (dob 14.6.09)

Leonie has been with us receiving short-term care for three weeks now with a view to becoming a permanent resident.

There will be an Assessment Meeting held on 9 September at which Mrs Green's social worker will be present. As Mrs Green's key worker I would be obliged if you could prepare a short written report about Leonie for the meeting.

Many thanks

Report writing

A report can be spoken or written. It can range from a very simple form-filling exercise on a pre-printed form to a complex, lengthy document containing terms of reference, an introduction, main body of the report, conclusion and recommendations. Below are some examples of occasions when an oral report might be required and when a written report might be needed.

Oral reports	*Written reports*
At a meeting or case conference	Accident report form
Report back to other staff on patients at a changeover of shift	Observations on a client
In a court of law	Observations on a patient who is being nursed in a special way
News report	Report on the type of bath which should be purchased for the use of clients with a physical disability

To do Add some other examples to these lists. Give examples from outside the care sector.

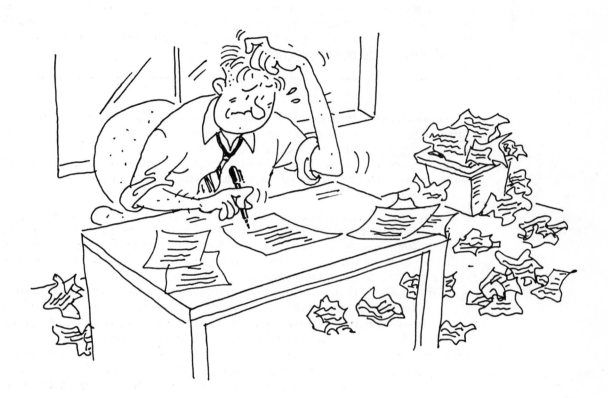

Here are some pointers to remember when writing a more complex report.

- A report is a factual document.
- It sets out to clarify a situation or solve a problem.
- One is usually asked to write a report by a colleague or colleagues in response to a situation or problem which may have arisen within the organisation.
- It may be necessary to interview colleagues within the organisation in order to write the report.
- A report is a formal piece of communication like a letter and should be written in clear, precise language using formal conventions of spelling, paragraphing, grammar and punctuation.
- The style should be impersonal and unbiased. It should not express personal opinion. For example, 'I think the Parker bath would be best because . . . ' but 'The Parker bath would be best because . . . '.

101

- Reports should be clear and easy to read so use headings, sub-headings and numbered points to display the material.

To do

Either at work or when you are on work experience from college ask your supervisor if you can have a copy of an accident report form. Imagine that one of your residents/patients has fallen down some steps and broken an ankle. Complete the necessary form so that you will know what to do another time.

It is important to remember that all kinds of reports, whether formal or informal, should be as objective as possible and if you need to express personal opinions this should be expressed in your 'Conclusion' section. Longer reports may have a formalised layout using prescribed headings and below is an outline of some of the terms which may be used.

Layout of formal reports

- *Title page* – should indicate the title of the report, the author's name, who has requested the report to be written and the date it was written.
- *Introduction* – this is used to outline the terms of reference of the report. These indicate the subject matter to be investigated and the report must not go outside these boundaries.
- *Main body* – this considers, in depth, the issues identified in the introduction. It also explains how the information was gathers, for example who has been interviewed. Headings and numbered points should be used in this section in order to make material clear.
- *Summary* – only necessary if the report is very long. Summarises briefly the ground covered and states whether the objectives have been achieved or not. The summary enables the reader to grasp the main points without necessarily reading the whole of the report.
- *Recommendations* – states how, in the opinion of the writer(s), the matter may or may not be resolved.
- *Appendices* – sometimes it is necessary to include further information like tables, graphs, drawings etc. which should be placed at the end of the report.
- *Index* – only necessary if the report is very long.

Non-verbal communication

This topic will be considered in more depth in Chapter 7, but it is vital to remember that when speaking or listening to a client, patient, other professional or just a friend you are also using non-verbal communication which reinforces, in a positive or negative way, what you are saying.

Speaking and listening skills

One fact is certain and that is that you will need to develop excellent listening and speaking skills in the caring professions, and be aware of the non-verbal messages that you are sending out. Outlined below is a summary of situations when you will need to call on these skills:

- welcoming a patient/client to the care setting;
- listening to and solving clients'/patients' problems;
- speaking and listening to colleagues;
- speaking and listening to other professionals, e.g. district nurse, doctor, social worker;
- solving your own personal problems at work;
- taking telephone calls and messages;
- attending a wide range of meetings, e.g. case conferences, staff meetings, assessment meetings;
- speaking and listening to other team members;
- speaking and listening to your 'boss'.

The list goes on and you should be able to think of plenty of other examples. Now we will examine how well you listen to what your friends and other people say to you. Many people think they are good listeners but there is a difference between just listening and active listening.

Active listening

You listen well when:

- you are interested;
- you are familiar with the speaker and subject;
- when the language is clear;
- when you are comfortable and relaxed;
- when there aren't many distractions.

To do

In pairs take it in turns to talk to your friend about something which has happened to you this week. Time this for two minutes. Now the listener should try to summarise what was said. How accurate was it? Now swap roles.

Successful listening does not just happen. Actually absorbing what is being said requires concentrated effort and active listening. You can achieve this by doing the following.

- *Focusing* on what the person is saying. Clear your mind of trivia and listen to what is being said even if you think you will not like it. By adopting a state of lively curiosity you will become more attentive to what is being said.

- *Identify* the essentials of the communication:
  — Who is the speaker?
  — What is the speaker saying? It is vital to identify the main threads of an argument.
  — Why is the speaker speaking? Are they worried or upset, being persuasive or just giving information?
  — How effectively is the speaker speaking? Are they using the conventions of speech and body language in order to get their message across?
- *React* – remember that communication is a two-way process. Feedback stimulates your awareness of what is being said and makes you ask questions. It also motivates you to listen.
- *Combine* all the information so that it becomes a secure package in your mind. Relate this new information to any other which you may have on the same topic. How does new material fit into what you already know? Do you need to modify your opinion? Have you learnt anything new from listening this time?

To do

Having read the advice on active listening above, repeat the two-minute listening exercise using different material with a friend. Can you remember more points this time? Do you now understand the difference between listening and active listening?

Speaking skills

In many of the situations that we identified at the beginning of this section you will be listening and then speaking in turn. Speech is a very important when working with patients/clients on a one-to-one basis. Probably 25 per cent of your time at work is spent using oral communication as a tool.

Perhaps the situation that people find most difficult is when they are asked to speak at a meeting in front of more senior colleagues and the words just don't come out the way you wanted them to. There are ways in which you can improve your oral communication, so let's consider some tips.

- *Audibility* – make sure people can hear what you are saying. Modify this to the situation in which you find yourself.
- *Pace* – if you are at a meeting try to pace your speech. Sometimes because people are nervous they speak too quickly.
- *Pitch* – this is the up and down element in your voice, so when you are speaking at a meeting try to vary this. It helps to keep colleagues interested in what you are saying.
- *Stress and emphasis* – you can stress certain words when you are speaking to hammer the point home.
- *Tone* – do think about the tone of your voice. Are you speaking in a pleasant way, a bullying way or a haughty way? This will affect how people receive your message.

- *Organise* – make sure if you are at a meeting that you have thought out clearly in your own mind what you are going to say before you open your mouth. If you have to make a lengthy contribution at a meeting make some notes to take into the meeting with you.

To do

Prepare a three-minute talk on a topic of your own choosing for the rest of the group. You may use notes. Video the talks, then watch them and make constructive and helpful comments on each one using the above headings.

Here are some specific situations where you will have to combine and use the different skills we have been considering.

Welcoming clients/ patients

You need to remember that when you are welcoming a new patient or client to your particular care setting, whether it is a day or residential setting, that they are likely to be feeling more nervous than you are. Remember that you are already familiar with the daily routine and the surroundings. Imagine what it would feel like to be an old person coming into a residential home for the first time, leaving behind your home, belongings, friends and familiar

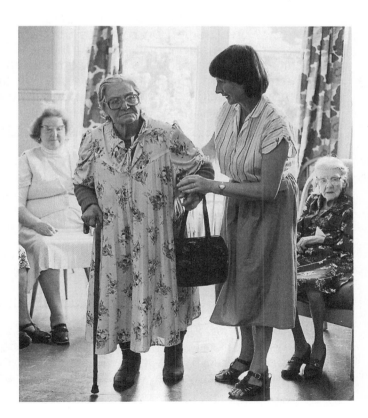

surroundings. Not very easy. Or imagine someone coming on to your hospital ward who has perhaps never been into hospital before. A daunting experience indeed, seeing all those nurses, doctors and other professionals in different uniforms and not understanding exactly who they are. So how can you as a carer make your client's welcome a bit more special?

You can try the following.

- Recognise that each client is an individual human being and unique.
- Welcome them and their relatives or friends warmly.
- Use positive body language and above all smile.
- Shake their hand, and state clearly your name and position within the organisation. Be sensitive to their mood and plan your communication accordingly.
- Don't be shy – have something to say – talk to them about their journey or ask them a few questions about themselves.
- Listen actively to what they are saying.

If you can think about welcoming a new patient/client in this way, even if you are not feeling particularly happy yourself, then you will have conducted yourself in a professional manner and not have let your inner feelings show.

To do

Work in groups of three and take it in turns to carry out a role play. One of you is an observer. One of you is a patient who is coming into hospital for a routine operation, the other is the nurse on duty when the patient arrives and whose job it is to welcome them on to the ward. Change the roles round until all three have had an attempt at each role. The observer should particularly focus and comment on the use of body language, speaking and listening skills.

Attending meetings

As part of your role in working as a carer it is likely that you will be required to attend and take part in a range of different types of meeting, for example case conferences, staff meetings, reviews of client's/patient's progress and client/patient assessment meetings. As a carer you may be responsible for speaking on behalf of another client/patient, which is a big responsibility, so you need to consider how you can be as effective as possible in a meeting. Many people find meetings a little threatening, but if you can develop a few basic skills you can make things easier for yourself.

To do

When you are out on work experience or at work ask if you can attend a meeting purely as an observer. Take notice of how well or otherwise people speak. Ask yourself whether or not they went to the meeting well prepared. Did they actively listen to other people's points of view?

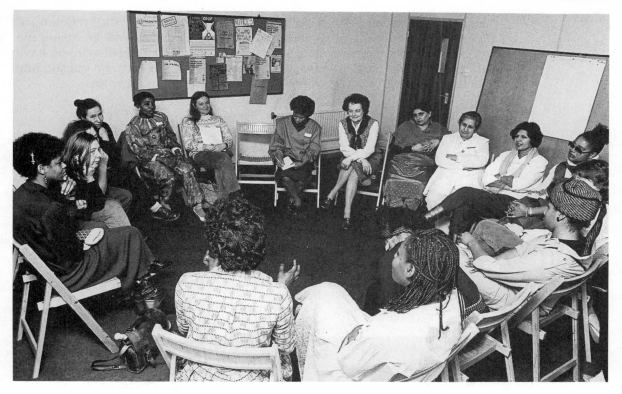

Here are a few tips which may assist you when you have to take part in a meeting:

- Don't go to a meeting badly prepared. Always take a copy of the agenda and any other documents which you might need, e.g. patient/client records.
- If you know you are going to have to speak about a topic make some supporting notes before you go into the meeting.
- When you have to contribute, speak clearly, in a good tone and maintain eye contact. Don't talk to the floor!
- Listen actively to what other people are saying, and modify your thoughts and opinions if necessary in the light of what is being said. Make a few written notes when other people are speaking. This can act as a memory jogger if you need to contribute later on.
- Make sure you get a copy of the minutes of the meeting and act on anything which you have been designated to carry out.

Telephone technique

When working in a care setting, whether community or residential, it is very likely that you may be speaking on the phone to members of the general public and other professionals, as well as patients, clients and their relatives. One important thing to remember when using the telephone is that it is one form of communication where you cannot see the other person. In a

107

face-to-face conversation people use non-verbal communication to reinforce what they are saying, e.g. nods, smiles etc., but when you are using the phone you can't see the other person so in order to get feedback you have to rely on using paralanguage, e.g. grunts, aah!, mmm! etc. and questioning techniques which can be difficult to master. Here are a few tips.

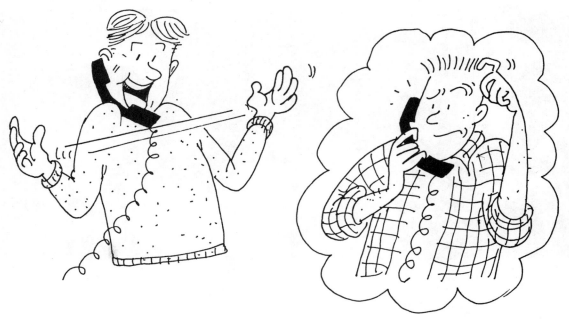

'It was this big!'

Answering the telephone

When answering the telephone always be polite, cheerful and efficient.

BEFORE:

- Make sure you get to know your telephone system. For example, learn how to transfer a caller efficiently.
- Always keep a pen and pad by the telephone.
- Stop talking to other people and reduce noise in your immediate environment.
- Announce the name of the organisation (not necessary if call has come via an operator), your name, ward/section and position.
- Be willing to try and answer any query.

DURING:

- If the message involves names and addresses or figures which are not clear read them back to the caller or ask them to spell them.
- Give continuance messages to caller, e.g. 'Go on'.

- Don't ask caller to 'hold on' while trying to sort out a query. Offer to call them back.
- If it is a lengthy message, summarise the main points to the caller before you put the phone down.
- Agree what happens next.

AFTER:

- Make sure you understand your notes.
- Act on the notes immediately, e.g. write them down in your diary.
- If you have taken a message for someone else put the date and time of the call on the message and leave it somewhere prominent so the person will find it, for example in the centre of their desk or in their tray where their mail and correspondence is left.

Making a telephone call

BEFORE:

- Keep in mind the purpose of your call.
- Make notes of facts, dates etc. to which you may need to refer.
- Have beside you client/patient records that you may need to refer to during the conversation.
- Have a pad and pen ready for your notes.
- Know who you want to speak to.
- Remember there are times when calls are cheaper. Can your call wait?
- Dial your number accurately, especially if it is long distance.

DURING:

- Give an appropriate greeting, e.g. 'Good morning', state your name and organisation, and who you want to speak to.
- Keep you call brief and to the point.
- State your subject clearly to put the recipient in the picture.
- Refer periodically to your own notes.
- Pause occasionally to get feedback to check that your message is being understood.
- Spell names and addresses. Repeat any numbers.
- Summarise the main points of a long conversation.
- If you have to leave a message for someone else help the person who answered the phone to get the right message.

AFTER:

- Add anything essential to your notes.
- Date the note.
- Take any action necessary as a result of the call, e.g. make a note on a patient's record, or put a date in your diary.
- Pass on the results of your call to anyone else concerned with the matter.

Key points

- Verbal, written and non-verbal communication skills are all vital skills in the business of caring.
- You may work with client groups, for example visually or hearing impaired people, or people with special learning needs who may find it difficult to communicate for a range of reasons. They will need to develop other means of communicating with you, for example touch.
- The formal written skills of letter, memo and report writing are important. Pay particular attention to tone, layout, paragraphing, spelling and grammar.
- Speaking and listening skills are equally important. *Remember active listening*, which means that you absorb what people are saying to you by shutting out external distractions.
- Twenty-five per cent of your time at work is spent using speaking and listening skills.
- Develop a positive approach when welcoming new clients to the care setting by using a combination of verbal and non-verbal communication.
- Develop a good telephone technique. Remember, you cannot see the other person, so you need to use paralanguage and other questioning techniques in order to get feedback.
- Communication skills can be developed and improved throughout life and by doing so you will have the satisfaction of knowing that you are communicating effectively and professionally with your clients/patients.

7 *Interpersonal skills*

Interpersonal communication describes the face-to-face communication which you have with people, both at work and socially, in your day-to-day life. It therefore includes non-verbal communication as well as the spoken word. Interpersonal communication is usually referred to in the context of one person relating to another, but of course in our daily lives we often find ourselves interrelating in small groups or large groups and with more than one person.

In the previous chapter we considered briefly how non-verbal communication interacting with our speaking and listening skills can affect the meaning of what we are saying. It can also affect the way in which another person receives and interprets the message.

In this chapter we are going to examine the nature of interpersonal skills, and some ways in which you can build on and improve your own skills.

Body language

Body language can tell us a considerable amount about people's attitudes, thoughts and feelings. For example, an actor on stage uses non-verbal communication, combined with the spoken word, to portray the character he or she is playing. An absent-minded professor might be portrayed by the actor wearing a wild wig, thick glasses, an old, baggy, tweed suit, and by taking on the persona and gestures of the character. Similarly, in real life we play different roles and use non-verbal communication to reinforce these roles in the same way.

By becoming more aware and controlling the non-verbal communication which we use we can become more effective in our relationships with other people. In other words, communication skills are learnt, not instinctive, and it is possible to learn more in order to get on better with people.

The elements of body language

There are seven main elements to body language. These are:

- gesture;
- expression;
- body posture;
- body space and proximity;
- touch;

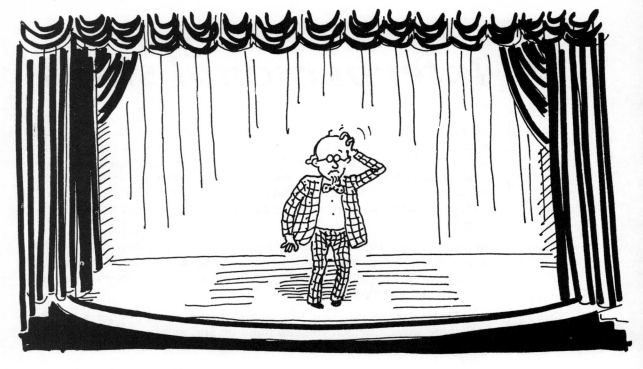

'Where's the audience gone?'

- reinforcement activity (paralanguage);
- dress.

Gesture

This is the way in which we use our hands and arms to express ourselves. We often use gestures when we are talking to a group of people, or are describing a particular object or giving directions to someone. There are whole languages which rely on gesture alone, for example sign language for hearing-impaired people or for use with hearing-impaired people without speech.

Expression

This is the way we use our faces to say something about the way we are feeling, for example whether we are bored, happy or sad. These are the kinds of signs we look for when meeting a person for the first time.

For example, when you meet a client/patient for the first time, by observing some of these facial expressions, you can begin to learn something about how that person is feeling even before they begin to speak.

Eye contact can also come into this category. If two people have a lot of eye contact it can mean that they have a trusting relationship. If someone you do not know has a lot of eye contact with you it can be a very uncomfortable experience, for example at a job interview. It's good to maintain eye contact but not to eyeball somebody!

Body posture

This the way in which we hold our bodies. If you can demonstrate a relaxed posture when you are dealing with a work colleague, for example, it indicates to the other person that you have confidence in them. However, it would be inappropriate to assume a very relaxed body posture at a job interview because this might indicate to the interviewer a lack of concentration and interest in the job. It is probably equally as bad at a job interview to sit with tightly crossed arms, as this can indicate a very closed and tense attitude to the interviewer.

Body space and body proximity

This phrase describes how close we stand or sit to other people. People need a certain amount of space around them in order to feel comfortable. Body space will also be affected by formal and informal situations, and whether the interaction is with a male or a female and perhaps the age of a person. In your interaction with clients and patients you should consider the factor of space carefully. If you are listening to someone's problem you should not sit so close to the other person that your knees are almost touching, since this may invade the other person's body space. Placing the chairs at right angles to one another is quite a good idea.

People often judge status by body proximity, so while it may be all right to be close to a friend, it may be unacceptable to be too close to the boss in a more formal setting. It may be considered that you are being too familiar.

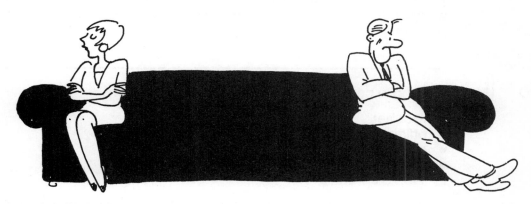

'I didn't want to talk to you anyway!'

Touch

This element is about who we touch, the way in which we touch people and how we touch them. Touch can give out a lot of signals about relationships, status and degrees of friendliness. For example, lovers will touch frequently and in a tender way. Women tend to be more tactile than men.

113

Touch can be a useful way of telling a client/patient that you care. For example, someone who has just been bereaved may not be able to speak about their loss but a reassuring touch can express that you care. Touch can also be reassuring to other kinds of client groups. For example, if a person is mentally ill, perhaps depressed, and is finding it difficult to talk about how they are feeling, then touch again can show that you care.

However, as carers we also need to be very aware of gender issues and the problems that touch can cause. For example, a male care worker working in an observation and assessment centre with young male and female teenagers would need to be very careful about touch, because it could so easily be misinterpreted. As a general rule it is probably better to avoid touch in this kind of situation. There is a fine dividing line between caring and professionalism, and it is important that carers act in a professional manner.

Similarly, if you have to discipline a young person, it is important that you follow any guidelines which are laid down by your organisation and to ensure that another member of staff is present so that there is a witness to whatever you say or do in carrying out the discipline.

Reinforcement activity (para-language)

This describes the non-verbal signs which can accompany speech. For example, grunts of approval about what a person is saying or a nod of the head, or an interested look can all indicate to another person that they should continue with what they are saying and that you are interested. This is obviously an important factor in any client/patient relationship.

Dress

This element covers the image which we present to the world. The clothes we wear, the hairstyle we have and the make-up we use all say something about the kind of person we are.

To do

Working in pairs consider the following occupations

- teacher;
- office worker;
- officer in charge of an old people's home;
- social worker;
- shop assistant.

Describe the clothes you would expect them to wear for work and at home. Compare your results with those of another pair. Do your stereotypes match?

Speech

Speech is the other main tool of interpersonal communication. Just as non-verbal communication is a language composed of signs, so is speech.

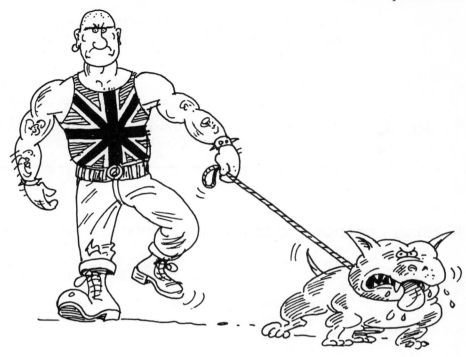

The way we dress says something about the kind of person we are.

We learn to speak a language at an early age because it enables us to satisfy many of our basic human needs.

Both verbal language and non-verbal communication are linked to culture. Non-verbal gestures and expressions mean different things in different cultures. For example, men from Middle Eastern cultures like to stand close and face the person they are talking to, but many men from Western cultures would not be used to this kind of approach and would shy away from it. Men from some of the Mediterranean countries like Italy, Greece and Turkey will often embrace one another and kiss on the cheeks. Many men in the UK would find that unacceptable.

Speech is also a part of our culture. Many words mean different things to people from other countries. For example, many English words have a different meaning to an American. Sometimes words from one language do not translate easily into another because spoken language develops and expresses ideas which our culture believes in. And sometimes languages borrow words from other languages because they do not have suitable ones of their own. For example, the French language includes words like *'le*

115

weekend' and 'le camping' which are borrowed from the English language, and the English have borrowed words like cul-de-sac and discothèque from the French.

To do

As a group give some other examples of the ways in which non-verbal communication can mean different things in other cultures.

Making contact and forming relationships with others

There are certain strategies and skills which we can adopt in order to help us get on better with other people. These are:

- being able to present oneself effectively;
- being able to perceive oneself and others effectively;
- being able to empathise with others;
- being able to respond positively to feedback;
- being able to listen effectively.

Presentation of self

Because we all play different roles in our lives we present different personalities to different people according to the situation in which we find ourselves. For example if you work as a nursing assistant you would present a caring a professional approach to your patients. In other words you would use the language and non-verbal communication which was appropriate to that situation. However, if you were going out for a drink after work with some friends, male and female, your self-presentation would be completely different because you might perhaps fancy someone in the group. This changing of roles is not something which we do consciously, but we need to be aware that we present different personae, depending on the situations in which we find ourselves. In other words the role in which we find ourselves shapes our use of language and non-verbal communication.

Perception of self and others

The two main aspects to the way we see ourselves are:

- our own self-image and
- our own self-esteem.

Self-image describes how we see ourselves as physical human beings and the kind of personality we think we have. For example, we may think we are too fat or too thin or we may not like the colour of our hair, but personality traits affect the way we interact with other people more than our appearance.

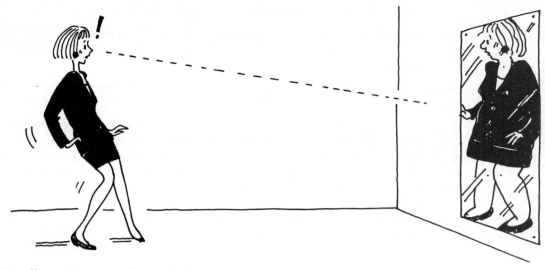

'I really must go on a diet again!'

Our own self-image is developed and shaped by our relationships with others. However, other people never see us as we see ourselves. For example, a person with a physical disability may have a rather negative self-image because some people may view physically disabled people in a negative light and this serves to reinforce the person's opinion about themselves. It is important to try to view our personality and personal qualities in a positive light, because if we do we are more likely to be positive in our relationships with other people.

Most people also have an *ideal self-image* which involves an image of ourselves (or our families) as we would like to be in an ideal world. For example, parents may want their children to achieve certain successes in examinations at school, yet the child may not be able to achieve these goals. This can affect the child's personality and performance, and make an unhappy child.

Self-esteem

Self-esteem is the opinion which we have of ourselves. For example, you may feel that you are not particularly good at playing sport, but on the other hand you may be good at playing the guitar. If you can just shrug off the fact that you are not much good at sport, but that you have other qualities which make up for it then you are more likely to have a *positive self-esteem* and to view yourself in an objective light. In other words, if you develop a positive self-image and self-esteem it means you are likely to get on better with other people.

117

To do Ask a partner to list your positive personality traits. Now list your positive personality traits as you see them. Compare lists and see how different they are. Now reverse roles.

Perception of others

When meeting someone for the first time we can make assumptions, whether they are right or wrong, about the kind of person they are. Even before they speak their non-verbal language, as we have already seen, says something about the kind of person they are and how they are feeling on that particular day. So, how do we perceive others?

- *Personality* – we usually assess people in terms of a few traits. For example, we say they are outgoing, friendly or aggressive. So we build a picture of the person and this affects the way we communicate with them.
- *Emotion* – we use our perception skills and assess how someone is feeling. For example, if a person is feeling sad they may not want to listen to stories about the wonderful holiday that you have just had!
- *Attitude* – when communicating we try to see what the other person's attitude is towards us. Attitude affects the communication process. If we are warm and friendly then the other person is more likely to respond in a similar manner.
- *Knowledge and beliefs* – the knowledge and beliefs people have affect their relationships with others.
- *Assumptions* – we make guesses about someone's lifestyle, about the job they do and their background. For example, a person's job means that we may make an assumption about the social class to which they belong.

So our perception of other people is influenced by recognising non-verbal signals and by making assessments of them in terms of personality, emotion, their attitude to us, the knowledge and beliefs which they bring to a relationship, and assumptions which we have made. In other words we have a need to determine the kind of person we are dealing with and this in turn influences the way we will communicate with them. For example, a young person who is an offender may have a low self-esteem and it might be that by finding something that they can do well, like repairing motor bikes, you can build a more positive relationship with them and thus improve their self-esteem.

Problems with perception

There can be problems with judging someone on first impressions. For example, an elderly person in your care may be physically in very poor shape. This can affect your relationship with that person because you feel sorry for them, so you lose sight of the fact that they are an individual who has had an interesting life and may have a lot to contribute to your relationship.

It is important not to label people because this can also affect our relationships. For example, if we label a person as being aggressive this could cloud other people's perception of that person.

The worst kind of putting people in a category and labelling them is called *stereotyping*. This means that we use only a few simple signs like dress to place a person in a particular category.

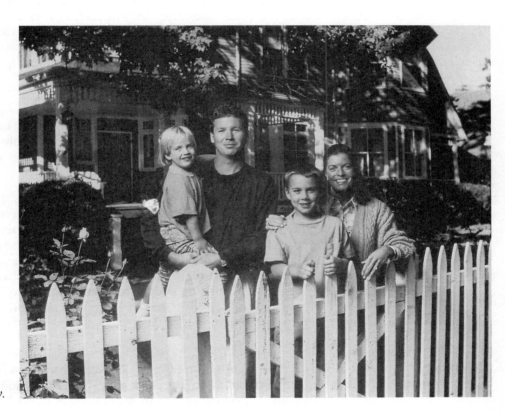

The media tend to present a 'stereotype' family.

The media are very good at doing this. An example of this would be the kind of advertisement where there is a typical family presented in order to sell the product. Mum stays at home in a lovely four-bedroom detached house with an exceptionally large kitchen, and she has two beautiful children and a loving husband. Do you get the picture? Most families do not live in this kind of way.

To do

As a group give examples of advertisements which use stereotyping as a means of selling their service or product. Why do they do this?

Empathy

Empathy can affect the way we build relationships and deal with other people, particularly when working in the caring field. It involves the ability to deal sensitively and sympathetically with another person, and to be able to 'put yourself in their place' and try to view the problem from their point of view.

For example, if you are dealing with an elderly person who has just entered residential care and they are feeling a sense of loss at having to leave their family, home and community they may be feeling very unhappy. If you can try to think how it might feel to be that person then it is likely that you will communicate with them in a more sensitive and understanding way. In the long term, if you are able to empathise in your relationships it is more likely that you will build an effective relationship.

Feedback

As we saw in Chapter 6 feedback refers to your ability to respond to the other person by using non-verbal communication, reinforcement activity and questioning techniques to indicate that you have understood and interpreted the message they are putting across.

If you are able to respond positively to feedback this can enhance the communication process. It doesn't mean that you have to agree with everything someone says, but if you are prepared to give them a fair hearing they are more likely to respond to you in a positive manner. For example, a client may want to tell you about an argument they have had with a friend. You may not agree with their point of view about the argument, but by listening and perhaps making suggestions you have shown that you value them as a person and are prepared to listen. In communication terms you have given them positive feedback.

Listening

We discussed the issue of listening in Chapter 6, but it is worth emphasising that it is very important to develop *active* listening skills, which means picking out the important points in a conversation, and working out the meaning and purpose of what the other person has to say. This means cutting out distractions, being aware of your own prejudices and not switching off from something you don't want to hear. All this requires considerable effort. It is about receiving the communication as well as giving it.

Clients'/patients' individuality

So far in this chapter we have considered how to try to build more positive relationships with people and some of the factors which can influence or get in the way of relationships. There are certain other individual factors which can also get in the way of effective personal relationships whether at work or home.

One of the basic tenets of the helping/counselling process is the need to recognise that every human being is a unique individual and that to try and help them we must accept them as they are and value them for themselves. In other words we must not try to impose our own values, beliefs, prejudices and standards on them. This is perhaps easier said than done and when communicating with patients/clients it can be very easy, through the use of non-verbal communication, the language that we use or our perception of others to indicate our non-acceptance or non-valuing of an individual.

Some of the individual factors which might affect relationships are:

- race;
- religion;
- age;
- gender;
- physical appearance;
- physical and mental ability.

An example of gender causing problems in a professional relationship might be that of a male care assistant being asked to bath a female patient. He is professionally competent to carry out this task but, understandably, the patient might object. If this is the case the patient's wishes should be respected in order to preserve the professional relationship between care assistant and patient.

A similar situation could occur if a female carer is asked to carry out a procedure which a male patient might feel embarrassed about.

For example, a young man might feel embarrassed about a female health care assistant being asked to shave and prepare him for an operation to remove his appendix. In this instance, if he prefers a male health care assistant to carry out the procedure, then his wishes should be respected.

Some care assistants who work with elderly people or disabled people talk to them in a very patronising way, particularly if the old person has Alzheimer's disease. This fails to recognise that person as an intelligent human being. It is important to look beyond the persona and realise that that person may have been a mother, had a career, and is loved and valued. They had a lot of life before they got Alzheimer's.

To do

Working in small groups of two or three and using your own personal experience, identify examples of how the above factors can get in the way of building relationships, whether personal or professional.

Clients'/patients' rights

There are certain basic human rights which should be accepted and acknowledged by all members of staff in any kind of care setting. These are:

- the right to confidentiality;
- the right to not be discriminated against on grounds of race, disability, age, gender and so on.

The right to confidentiality

As a member of a team of people working in a caring setting you will have access to personal files, whether written or stored on computer, which will contain private and personal information about the clients/patients in your care. Clients and patients will also, during the course of their conversations, tell you private and personal things about themselves and their family. For example, if you were counselling someone about their marital problems they might tell you about a sexual relationship that they had had outside of their marriage. This puts you, as the counsellor, in a very privileged position and the person has only told you this because they know you will keep that information to yourself.

It is therefore extremely important that you always respect this right and that, other than with you professional work colleagues, you do not divulge or discuss any of this information with anyone else. It is information which you are privileged to know about that person and if you divulge that information to an inappropriate person you are going to jeopardise your professional relationship with patient or client. The trust they had in you as a professional person will disappear immediately and once again your relationship with that person would be affected.

The right to non-discriminatory practices

People can be discriminated against for a variety of reasons including race, age, gender, sex, dress and so on. This discrimination can be evidenced in relationships with other people and it could be happening in your care setting.

An example of a patient/client being discriminated against could take the form of verbal abuse or threatening behaviour. If you have a client with severe learning difficulties who kept biting himself then a member of the care staff could threaten him verbally by telling him if he does that again he will not be allowed to take part in a certain outing which all the other residents are going on. There are clearly other ways of tackling this client's behaviour, but verbal threats are certainly not going to solve the problem. In fact they will only serve to stop the client and worker from establishing a more positive relationship.

A person living in a residential setting could be discriminated against because of the disability from which they suffer. For example, Parkinson's disease may make sufferers depressed and they may find it difficult to relate to people. It is quite likely that some members of care staff might find such patients difficult to deal with in terms of forming relationships and therefore avoid doing their share of caring or perhaps do not relate well to them when they do help to care.

In some instances specific residential provision is made for certain religious or ethnic groups, because they would perhaps find it more difficult to cope in a mixed setting. An example of this might be a home for elderly people who belong to a particular religion. There are some residential homes which cater specifically for ethnic minorities, but they tend to be few and far between.

If a resident from another culture has to live in a residential setting where they are in a minority it could mean that the staff do not understand the culture which the person belongs to and are not able to respond to their daily living needs or it could be that the person is forced to endure racist comments. With the Community Care Act in force from April 1993, local authorities may find it easier to make special provision for ethnic minority groups, because they are able to set up small units within residential homes for elderly people from ethnic minorities which will help to promote anti-discriminatory practice.

It is vital that care staff working in a residential setting, whether private, voluntary or statutory, have a forum in which they can raise discrimination issues without feeling uncomfortable. This is why regular staff meetings are absolutely essential. Care workers should be able to pass information back to management, as well as directives and policies being passed down to members of staff. Communication in any organisation should be a two-way process. It is still surprising how many care workers do not have access to regular staff meetings or a supervisor with whom they can discuss these issues.

To do

From your own personal experience give other examples of ways in which clients/patients have been discriminated against. How has it affected the client/patient relationship?

Working as a team member

So far we have discussed interpersonal relationships in terms of a one-to-one relationship, but in reality when you go on practical work experience from college or go to work you will be working with other people as part of a team and you will be part of a group relating perhaps to several people in differing situations. For example, you will encounter patient/client discussion groups, staff meetings, case conferences and so on. These people could be:

- colleagues working on a similar level in the organisation;
- managers or supervisors who are responsible for leading the team;
- clients or patients who are in your care.

A group at work can be described as a collection of people sharing some common purpose under a common leader, and seeing themselves as having a common identity.

The interpersonal techniques you will need to employ within a work group are essentially the same as those we have discussed earlier in this chapter, except that the multiple contacts you will be making ensure that the giving of feedback and the interpretation of non-verbal clues becomes even more important.

In a work team some sort of control by a leader is essential whether that leader is:

- chosen by the group,
- chosen for the group,
- or is self-appointed,

and no satisfactory interrelationship can take place without a leader.

A formal meeting is a good example of the difference between group and one-to-one interaction, because in a meeting the chairperson or group leader has to control the discussion. If everybody speaks at once there will be chaos. In a formal group meeting the leader has to control the discussion and the easiest way of doing this is for all the discussion to be channelled through the leader. In more informal groups a similar function arises as a natural group leader will emerge and that person will control the discussion in a more casual manner.

In a formal or an informal meeting the group leader has to be particularly adept at picking up non-verbal cues. It might be a partially open mouth or a raised finger, but only by picking up on these cues will the leader realise that somebody wishes to make a contribution.

To do

As a group watch a television discussion programme with the sound turned down. Jot down the kinds of non-verbal communication that are taking place in the group. If possible, video one of your group discussions at college and analyse the non-verbal cues taking place. Play the tape back with the sound turned down.

Interpersonal skills affect both our private and professional lives. These skills are about relationships and communicating in everyday life and it is vital to build on the skills you already have. They are skills which we all go on developing and improving throughout our lives, so keep on practising. Other people you relate to will be the ones who will benefit most, but you will also have the satisfaction of knowing that you are putting the utmost effort and skill into communicating effectively.

Key points

- Non-verbal communication (NVC) tells us a lot about other people's thoughts, feelings and attitudes.
- Positive NVC conveys interest, and adds warmth and sincerity to our relationships with other people.
- Self-image, self-esteem, our perception of others, our ability to respond to feedback and listen effectively are all factors which are important in establishing and maintaining good interpersonal relationships.
- Our perceptions of others are sometimes inaccurate. It is important to be aware of labelling and stereotyping.
- We need to value and respect people as individuals.
- We need to recognise and respect people's rights to such things as confidentiality and understand how this can affect personal relationships.
- At work we are members of a team interlinking with several people, and the same interpersonal skills and techniques apply equally to developing and maintaining relationships in this setting.
- Interpersonal skills can be developed, worked on and improved throughout our personal and professional lives. They are a very important skill!

8 Factors affecting development and behaviour

By the time children reach the age of eight they will already have made considerable developments, physically, intellectually and socially. This chapter and Chapter 9 will discuss these areas of development through from eight years to old age.

These two chapters will look at the factors that may affect the way individuals develop, and suggest reasons why some people develop differently from others. The normal developments usually follow a set pattern, but there may be some exceptions. These exceptions to the normal patterns may occur due to disabilities resulting in problems in certain areas, and these will be discussed in this chapter.

Factors influencing development and ageing

The ways that individual people grow and develop are governed by two main areas of influence, *genetic* and *environmental*. Genetic influences are those that are inherited from parents. Environmental influences are all other factors including physical, e.g. disease; intellectual, e.g. lack of stimulation; emotional, e.g. deprivation; and social factors, e.g. poor housing.

Genetic influences are passed on through genes, many thousands of which make up chromosomes. The ovum from the mother and the spermatazoa (or sperm) from the father each contain 23 chromosomes, and when the ovum and the sperm combine to form a single cell this cell then contains 23 paired chromosomes, giving a total of 46. This cell forms the blueprint for the new individual and each new cell in this individual will contain an identical set of chromosomes. Each gene in these chromosomes is responsible for a particular characteristic in the new individual. However, because each individual chromosome contains paired genes, one from the mother and one from the father, these may not be identical and the two paired genes may carry different instructions or messages.

For example in the genes carrying eye colour, one set of genes from the mother may carry blue colour, whereas the set from the father may carry brown colour. What colour eyes will the new individual have? The way that nature has solved this problem is by making some genes dominant and others recessive. This means that if the dominant gene is present then this is the characteristic that will show up in the new individual. Recessive characteristics will only appear in the new individual if there are recessive genes present from both parents. So, going back to the eye colour, the new individual is likely to have brown eyes as brown genes are dominant and blue genes are recessive. However, if both parents are brown eyed but carry a recessive blue eye gene some of their children may inherit two recessive genes and be blue eyed. Figure 8.1 shows how this may occur.

B = gene for brown eyes (dominant)
b = gene for blue eyes (recessive)

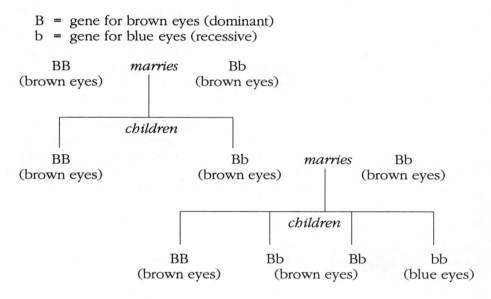

Figure 8.1 Genetic influences for eye colour

This demonstrates that if both parents have one dominant and one recessive gene each then there is a 1 in 4 chance that the children of brown-eyed parents will have blue eyes.

To do

Using the following chart find out within your group how many people have blue, brown or green eyes. Then find out the colour of their parents' eyes, if known. Draw bar charts to show the numbers of students with different eye colour to their parents, the numbers that have both parents with the same colour or with different colours. How many of the students have inherited the dominant colour, how many the recessive colour and how many have the same colour eyes as both of their parents?

Student eye colour	Parent 1 eye colour	Parent 2 eye colour	Student R, D or same as parents

It is thought that genetic influences play a part in determining many of an individual's characteristics. It is known that hair and eye colour, hair type, skin colour and facial bone structure are solely determined by genetics, while other characteristics such as height, weight and intellectual ability are probably influenced by both genetic and environmental factors. Many people believe that genetics determine the full potential of development, but the interactions of environmental factors determine how much of this potential is realised. For example, genetic influences may indicate that an individual has the potential to reach a height of 6 ft, but detrimental environmental factors may mean a height of only 5 ft 9 in is reached.

What are these environmental factors? They can be any external factor that has as effect on the development of the individual. If you think of all the different needs that an individual has, then deprivation of any of these can affect the way the person develops. It is normal practice to think of human needs under four headings (P.I.E.S):

- physical, e.g. food;
- intellectual, e.g. stimulation;
- emotional, e.g. love;
- social, e.g. a sense of belonging.

To do

As a group, think of all the needs that human beings have under the headings of physical, intellectual, emotional and social. Which specific areas of development do you think will be affected if these individual needs are not met?

In the rest of this chapter we are going to examine how deprivation in some of these areas may result in a failure to realise the full potential of the individual or may result in a disability.

Disabilities

In Chapter 1 a definition was given for disability, together with the different methods of classification. This section is going to look in more detail at some of the common disabilities and the effects they may have on development.

Congenital disabilities

Congenital disability is the term used to describe conditions that people are born with, and may be due both to genetic or environmental factors:

- *genetic factors* – those inherited on the genes from the parents;
- *environmental factors* – include injuries to the foetus while still in the uterus or injuries at birth.

Acquired disabilities

Acquired disabilities are due to injuries or illness after birth, or severe deprivation, whether physical or mental.

Sensory disabilities

There are two types of sensory disability:

- visual
- hearing.

Visual

The types of visual impairment are:

- blindness;
- partial sight; and
- refractive errors.

Blindness In the UK just over 100 000 people are registered as blind and a further 50 000 as partially sighted.

Blindness and partial sight can be caused by many different factors, both congenital and acquired. *Congenital blindness* may be due to:

- genetic factors;
- infections in the mother during pregnancy, such as rubella (German measles) or syphilis.

Acquired blindness may be caused by:

- tumours of the optic nerve;
- cataracts (misting of the lens of the eye);
- glaucoma (increased pressure in the eye);
- corneal ulcers;
- other conditions of the eye.

In most cases blindness cannot be cured, but partially-sighted people can sometimes be helped with the use of spectacles.

Refractive errors Refractive errors such as short and long sightedness (myopia and hypermetropia) are usually caused by the shape of the eyeball and are often determined genetically.

Both of these conditions can be rectified by the wearing of spectacles or contact lenses. These types of problem often change during a lifetime, or develop in later life, so it is important to receive regular eye tests.

Developmental issues Developmentally, sight problems may or may not cause problems. Much depends on early diagnosis and quick intervention. If children receive special help early enough they may develop quite normally and achieve their full potential. If help is not given at an early stage

129

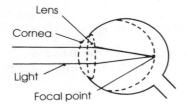

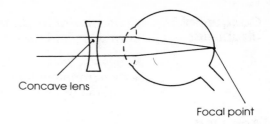

Concave lens

Focal point

Uncorrected myopia (short sightedness)

With uncorrected myopia, the images of distant objects are focused in front of the retina and appear blurred.

Corrected myopia

To see distant objects clearly, the power of the eye must be reduced by a concave lens.

How short sightedness is rectified by the wearing of glasses or contact lenses.

then there may be problems with intellectual, emotional and social development as children are deprived of normal stimulation and opportunities to communicate.

Refractory problems are the errors most likely to be missed and if they are overlooked the repercussions can be serious. If children develop either of these conditions, but more especially short sight, it may mean that they have difficulty seeing at school. This in turn may lead to learning difficulties as they miss out on a lot of information and they may be slower to complete their work.

To do

Construct a pie chart to illustrate how many people in your group suffer from short sight, long sight, other visual problems, and normal vision.

Hearing

The types of hearing impairment are:

- deafness;
- partial deafness;
- periodic deafness.

Congenital deafness affects about 1 in 10 000 people in the UK. Causes include:

- genetics;
- rubella during pregnancy;
- brain damage during birth.

Acquired deafness may be caused by:

- infections such as repeated ear infections or meningitis;
- accidental damage to the ears;
- senile deafness in older people as part of the ageing process.

There is usually no cure for hearing impairment, but hearing aids may help with partial deafness.

Behind-the-ear (Post-aural)

This type has all the equipment in a small case worn behind the ear. They are less conspicuous than the body-worn type but are less powerful.

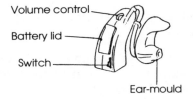

Body-worn

These are more powerful and have larger controls which are easier for arthritic people to manage. The case can be clipped to a pocket or the neck of a dress, and is connected to receiver and ear-mould by fine flex.

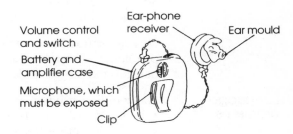

Types of hearing aid

Periodic deafness is usually due to infections either of the ear, sinuses or the adenoids (patches of lymph tissue at the back of the nose where it joins the mouth cavity). Treatment is usually successful and may involve treatment with antibiotics for the infections or surgery either to drain the middle ear or to remove the adenoids.

Developmental issues If hearing impairment is diagnosed at an early stage and specialised help provided, the child that is born with severe hearing impairment may develop normally in all major areas. Communication may be a problem, but many children are now taught to talk as well as to sign, and develop lip-reading skills in order to 'read' what the other person is saying. If hearing impairment is part of a greater problem associated with brain damage, then there may be more serious developmental problems which may affect all areas of development.

Periodic deafness needs to be detected early and it may be necessary for known victims to be tested on a regular basis. This condition is responsible for many early learning difficulties with young children, especially in the areas of communication. These include speech, reading and spelling. The repercussions of these problems may extend into children's later lives affecting some areas of schooling and education. Occasionally behavioural problems can result from hearing impairment, with the children either becoming withdrawn or aggressive as a reaction to their frustrations.

Speech

The types of speech disability are:

- stammering;
- language problems;
- cleft palate;
- dysphasia or breakdown of language;
- dysarthria or impaired speech formation;
- dysphonia or poor voice production.

131

Stammering

About 4 per cent of the population stammers, with males being affected more than females.

Although no one knows what actually causes someone to stammer, it is thought that emotional stress may act as a trigger.

Speech therapists can usually help with a variety of techniques that enable the individual to overcome the stammer.

Developmental issues Some people who stammer develop social problems through teasing and embarrassment, but with sympathetic handling all areas of development should be normal.

Language problems

Many children have speech problems while learning to talk, including the substitution of sounds, for example 't' for 'k', or they may leave out some sounds altogether. Most children will resolve these problems by the age of seven.

Sometimes if the child has suffered from hearing loss these problems may persist.

Speech therapy may be needed to overcome these problems. This treatment can also help in other speech disorders or speech development.

Developmental issues All other areas of development are usually normal and, with correct help, each child can reach their full potential.

Cleft lip and palate

Cleft lip is a vertical split in the upper lip, which may be a small notch or may extend to the nostrils. *Cleft palate* is when the two sides of the roof of the mouth or upper palate do not join before birth.

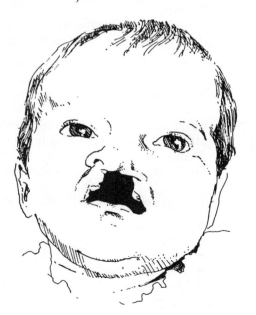

Cleft lip

About 1 in every 870 babies is born with one or both impairments. Although the cause is unknown, genetics may be involved as about one-third of those affected have relatives with one or both impairments.

The defects are usually detected at birth. In the case of cleft palate the baby is fitted with a plate to help with feeding before corrective surgery can take place, usually at about 18 months. Cleft lips are usually surgically repaired at about three months.

Speech therapy can help overcome any speech difficulties.

Developmental issues Once surgery and speech therapy have been given, development should not be affected. However, partial hearing impairment may also be present in cases of cleft palate, and some individuals may have other birth impairments,

Dysphasia or breakdown of language

In this case the parts of the brain that deal with the use of language are damaged and cannot control such things as recall of words or the ability to understand language. These people may know what things are used for, but may not be able to recall the correct word; or the person may speak freely, but the words do not make sense. This may also affect other methods of communication such as gestures and writing. Dysphasia is usually a result of brain injury often following a head injury or a stroke.

Speech therapy will endeavour to encourage memory and the relearning of the language.

Dysarthria or impaired speech formation

In this case the speech is slurred, volume uncontrolled with faulty rhythm and intonation. This condition is due to brain or nerve damage activating the muscles that control breathing, lips, tongue or palate, and leading to lack of co-ordination.

The causes of dysarthria are brain damage or nervous disorders such as Parkinson's disease.

Once again a speech therapist may be able to help or, if the condition if very severe, electronic communicators can be used. These display typed words on a screen, so communication may be slow.

Dysphonia or poor voice production

With dysphonia the voice alters in its quality. It may become weak, hoarse, nasal or become uncontrollable in pitch or volume.

Causes includes misuse of the voice, emotional problems, growths or paralysis of the vocal cords.

Misuse and emotional problems are usually temporary and the voice returns to normal when the cause disappears, but some speech therapy may be needed.

Tumours or growths can be removed surgically, although in the case of malignant (cancerous) tumours the whole larynx or voice box may have to be removed. In these cases the patients will have to learn to speak using the oesophagus instead, perhaps with the help of a vibrator.

Paralysis of the vocal cords may be congenital, or caused by an accident or disease. Most cases can be helped either by surgery or speech therapy.

To do

Find out what facilities are provided in your locality for:

a) detecting hearing and speech problems;

b) treating hearing and speech problems;

c) providing support for people with hearing and speech problems, and/or their relatives.

Autism

From the age of a few months an autistic child does not relate to others, but lives in a world of its own. Frequently they have little or no speech, resent change and can only learn to play repetitive games.

This is a fairly rare condition, affecting about 2 to 4 children in every 10 000. Autism is a condition which affects three times more boys than girls.

The precise cause is unknown, although some cases are associated with brain damage.

Children with autism require specialist help, including schooling and sometimes behaviour therapy. Parents need support and counselling.

Developmental issues If detected early and treated, usually in special schools, children with autism may be able to show some normal developments, and take part in normal adult life in later years. However, many require special, and often residential, care throughout life.

Dyslexia

This condition is sometimes referred to as word blindness, as sufferers have difficulties with reading. Ninety per cent of people diagnosed with dyslexia are male.

The cause of dyslexia is unknown, although recent research provides evidence that it is an inherited neurological disorder.

Developmental issues In all other aspects of development and behaviour the child is normal, but just has severe difficulties with reading and spelling. If the problem is not diagnosed early the child can become frustrated and may have behavioural or other learning problems as a result. Early treatment by remedial teachers can help the child to overcome the problems by 'tricks', and they go on to lead successful lives.

Cerebral palsy

This is a condition that is caused by brain damage either at or after birth. There are three types:

- *spastic* – unable to relax muscles;
- *athetoid* – unable to control movement;
- *ataxic* – poor co-ordination and balance.

At birth cerebral palsy is caused by lack of oxygen or bleeding into the brain; after birth it is due to jaundice, injury or convulsions. It is usually detected at birth or soon after, and can vary from very mild to very severe, depending how much brain damage has occurred. This condition may be accompanied by other conditions such as hearing impairment or epilepsy, and the individual may range from having low intelligence to very high intelligence, with some completing university education.

Individuals with cerebral palsy need early assessment and appropriate treatment, which includes physiotherapy, hydrotherapy, speech therapy and conductive therapy. With encouragement and long treatments many individuals can overcome some of their problems and lead full lives, while others will need to be in a care environment for most of their lives, often in specialist centres.

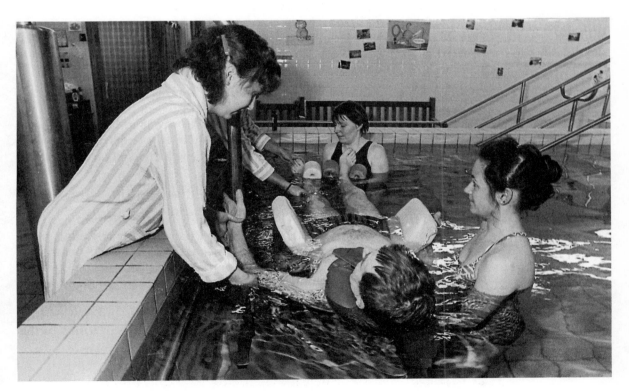

The hydrotherapy pool at St Thomas's Hospital, London.

To do

In small groups, find out as much as you can about physiotherapy, hydrotherapy, speech therapy, conductive therapy. Present short seminars to the whole group.

Spina bifida

The literal translation of this is 'split spine' and the condition means that the bones and other tissues surrounding the spinal cord do not form properly, leaving the nerves and membranes exposed. In the UK about 40 per 100 000 babies are born with this condition, which is congenital and appears to run in families, although the cause is not known. The severity of the condition can vary from mild, showing no external signs or symptoms, to severe, including brain damage, hydrocephalus (water on the brain) and paralysis.

In mild cases no treatment is necessary, but in severe cases surgical correction will be carried out soon after birth.

Developmental issues The future development of the child will depend on the severity of the damage and the success of the surgery. Intellectual development can be completely normal if there is no brain damage. Physical development will be affected if there is weakness or paralysis due to damaged nerves in the spinal cord. In severe cases the person may need to be cared for in a specialist centre.

Hydro-cephalus

Literally 'water on the brain', this condition results in an abnormally enlarged head, due to an excessive build-up of cerebro-spinal fluid, the fluid that surrounds the brain.

Hydrocephalus is caused when the circulation of this fluid is blocked, or if the fluid is produced in over-large quantities. If present at birth it is usually associated with spina bifida. This condition can occur in later life, due to meningitis or a brain tumour. In these cases there is no enlargement of the head as the skull bones will have fused, resulting in increased pressure inside the skull causing headache and vomiting.

The only treatment for this condition is surgical, introducing a tube with a valve, to drain the fluid away into the bloodstream.

If this treatment is carried out early, before there is any resulting brain damage, then development should be normal. If the condition is not treated or if there is a delay in treatment the person may suffer from brain damage, blindness or spasticity, with the associated effects on development.

Muscular dystrophy

This is a genetic disorder in which there is a slow but progressive degeneration of the muscle tissues. There are many different forms of this condition:

* Duchenne;
* Becker's;
* myotonic;

- limb-girdle;
- facioscapulohumeral.

Duchenne

This is the most common and most severe type of muscular dystrophy, affecting about 1 in 3000 boys.

It is inherited through a recessive, sex-linked gene so that only males are affected and only females can pass it on. The condition is usually diagnosed by the age of three when the young boys do not reach the normal physical milestones of development.

Developmental issues

Although many boys learn to walk, many of them are wheelchair users by the age of 12, due to deterioration of the muscles. Most boys do not survive beyond their teenage years, usually dying from heart failure or chest infections. There is no cure, but better care results in longer life spans, and some boys can achieve well academically, providing they do not miss too much schooling.

Becker's

This condition produces similar symptoms as the Duchenne type, but does not start until later in childhood. The rate of deterioration is much slower with many of the sufferers reaching their 50s. It is also a sex-linked genetic disorder.

Myotonic

This form affects the muscles of the hands and feet, with the muscles contracting strongly, but not relaxing easily. This condition is associated with the development of cateracts in middle age, with baldness, mental impairment and endocrine disorders.

Limb-girdle

This can take different forms, but mainly affects the hip and shoulder muscles. It can start in late childhood or early adulthood and progression is slow.

Facioscapulo-humeral

This form can develop any time between the ages of 10 and 40 years. It only affects the muscles of the face, shoulders and upper arm. Progression is slow and severe disability is rare.

Multiple sclerosis

This is a progressive condition affecting the nervous system, in which the protective coverings (myelin sheath) of the nerves in the brain and spinal cord are destroyed. Symptoms range from tingling and numbness through the paralysis. Typically, there is a patchy pattern of disabilities, variable in site and time, often with unpredictable improvements.

Multiple sclerosis is five times more common in temperate climates such as Europe and the USA, with about 1 in every 1000 people being affected. It is the most common acquired disease of the nervous system in young adults.

The cause remains unknown, although it is thought to have some genetic factor as relatives of affected people are eight times more likely than others to get the condition.

There is no cure for multiple sclerosis and little treatment that has more than a slight benefit to most sufferers. Some find that modifications to their diet, or taking evening primrose or sunflower oils help. Hyperbaric oxygen treatment (high-pressure oxygen chambers) has also been tried.

The usual advice to people is to live as active a life as their disabilities allow, and to treat symptoms as they appear, for example using physiotherapy to help weakened muscle groups.

Developmental issues Until the symptoms appear in young or later adulthood, all aspects of development are normal. The effects of the disease vary from time to time and from person to person, so disabilities will depend on the way the disease develops. Common effects are:

- disturbances to vision;
- weakness and lack of use of some muscle groups, affecting movement;
- lack of co-ordination and loss of balance;
- numbness, and feelings of pins and needles;
- incontinence.

Haemophilia

This is a bleeding disorder. In haemophilia there is a lack of a clotting factor known as factor VIII, and the disease can vary in intensity. Most bleeding episodes involve bleeding into joints and muscles which can be extremely painful. Haemophilia affects about 1 male in 10 000.

This condition is due to a defective gene which is passed through females and affects males.

Modern treatment involves the controlling of bleeding by infusions of concentrated factor VIII, which has improved the quality of life considerably.

Developmental issues Physical development may be affected by limitations due to joint damage. However many boys have no developmental problems at all. Sufferers are still advised to avoid sports and occupations that involve risk of injury, otherwise they can participate fully in all aspects of life. One sad side-effect has been the transmission of the HIV (Aids) virus during treatments with contaminated blood products before the connection between blood products and HIV was recognised, and some boys with haemophilia have had positive HIV tests. This may, of course, affect their life expectancy.

Sickle cell anaemia

The red blood cells of affected people contain an abnormal type of haemoglobin (the oxygen carrying pigment), called haemoglobin S. When there is a shortage of oxygen, for example following exercise or chest infections, the haemoglobin S crystallises and the cells distort into a sickle shape. This leads to a severe form of anaemia. These abnormal cells are unable to pass through tiny blood vessels, causing blockages and damage to various organs. These incidents are called sickle cell crises.

People suffering from this condition are more prone to infections such as pneumonia and septicaemia. If the blocking of blood vessels occurs in the brain, then brain damage can result in fits or a stroke.

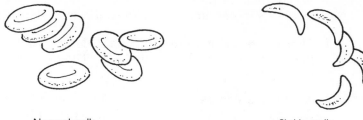

Normal cells　　　　　　　　　　　Sickle cells

Black people are more commonly affected with sickle cell anaemia, with people from Mediterranean origins less commonly affected. In the UK about 1 in 150 Afro-Caribbeans is affected.

Sickle cell anaemia occurs in individuals who have inherited haemoglobin S from both parents. If it is inherited from one parent only, the person will have a sickle cell trait, but is usually free from symptoms. However, if two people with the trait have children, then there is a one in four chance of the children having sickle cell anaemia, a two in four chance of them having the trait, and a one in four chance that the child will have neither. Anyone with relatives having sickle cell anaemia are advised to have tests to determine whether they are a carrier, and before having children carriers should obtain genetic counselling.

There is no cure for this condition. Life-long treatment with folic acid is given for the anaemia, and antibiotics and immunisations are given to protect against infection. During crises blood transfusions, oxygen therapy and pain-killing drugs are given, depending on the symptoms and the severity of the crises.

Developmental issues　Mortality is still high in the under fives, although improvements in treatment have enabled more people to survive into adulthood. Physical exercise is often limited because of the dangers of physical exertion. Cognitive development can be normal providing there is no brain damage. Emotionally people with sickle cell anaemia and their families require a lot of support and counselling.

Heart disorders

The heart is a vital organ which never stops working until death, however there are a variety of disorders that can affect it:

- congenital defects;
- infection;
- impaired blood supply;
- drugs and poisoning.

Congenital defects

There are two common types of defect, *septal* and *valves*. Septal and valve defects can occur during the development of the heart in pregnancy. The defects may be due to drugs or rubella during the pregnancy, but in most cases the cause is unknown.

139

Today most of these defects can be repaired soon after birth with a high level of success, and normal development should follow.

Infections

These can result from congenital defects or as a complication of other infections such as rheumatic fever. They can result in malfunctions of the heart valves.

Antibiotics can be used in the treatment of infections, but the resulting damage may require surgical correction. Physical development may be restricted if the damage is severe.

Impaired blood supply

This affects the heart muscle and prevents the heart from operating normally. It is the major cause of heart disease in developed countries. The coronary arteries which supply the heart muscle become narrowed and parts of the muscle are deprived of oxygen. The person may then develop angina or have a heart attack which may affect the amount of physical activity that can be undertaken.

Drugs and poisoning

Many drugs used to treat other conditions can result in changes to the heart beat or damage the heart muscle. However, the most common type of poisoning to affect the heart is alcohol. A large intake over many years can result in the heart becoming enlarged and heart failure developing. It is possible to recover from these conditions if the drugs or alcohol intake are stopped.

Epilepsy

Epilepsy is described as a condition in which there is an abnormal pattern of electrical activity in the brain, resulting in fits or seizures.

In the majority of cases the first incident usually occurs in childhood or adolescence. There are two main types:

- *grand mal* or major fits;
- *petit mal* or absence fits.

During a *grand mal* attack the person usually falls down unconscious and has severe muscle spasms. On recovery the person may have headaches, loss of memory and some confusion. During a *petit mal* or absence fit the person, usually a child, has a momentary loss of consciousness without abnormal movements. To an onlooker it may appear that the person is just day-dreaming, or no one may notice the incident.

This is a condition which affects about 1 in 200 people, and may result from brain damage or other diseases. Although in many cases there is no obvious cause, in others there appears to be an inherited tendency.

Epilepsy can be well controlled through the use of drugs and most treated epileptics can lead a full and normal life, with no developmental effects.

Developmental issues If there are frequent fits these can disrupt a child's learning processes and may lead to a failure in intellectual development. If the condition developed in early life the problem may decrease, with about one-third of children with epilepsy growing out of the condition during adolescence.

Coeliac disease

This is a condition in which the victims have a sensitivity to gluten, a protein found in wheat, rye and some other cereals.

The incidence in the UK is about 40 people in 100 000, but in parts of Ireland it is as high as 300 in 100 000. In Africa and Asia coeliac disease is extremely rare.

It is not known what causes the disease, but it seems to be more common in some families than in others.

Gluten damages the lining of the small intestine, thus causing malabsorption of nutrients which can result in anaemia and skin problems. If gluten is avoided in the diet then the symptoms soon clear up, but a gluten-free diet does mean avoiding all foods containing wheat, rye and barley such as bread, flour and cereals. This condition does not affect development if treated.

To do

Construct a weekly menu providing a balanced diet for someone suffering from coeliac disease.

Cystic fibrosis

Victims of this disease suffer from respiratory and digestive disorders due to the secretion of a sticky mucus which is unable to lubricate or flow freely in the nose, throat airways and intestines.

The incidence among Western Europeans and white Americans is about 1 in 2000, but is much lower in Asians and Afro-Caribbeans.

Cystic fibrosis is an inherited disease, being carried on defective, recessive genes, which means that a defective gene has to be received from both parents in order for the disease to develop.

Before the mid-1970s many people with cystic fibrosis died in childhood, but with drug treatments, including the use of antibiotics and physiotherapy, most now survive into adulthood.

Lung damage is often the result of repeated chronic chest infections, and malabsorption is also a problem.

Developmental issues The effects of the disease means that normal physical development may be affected, but psychological development is usually normal.

Skeletal disorders

These can include a number of conditions such as club foot or congenital dislocation of the hip, most of which are detected at birth and with early treatment there should be little or no impediment to development.

141

To do

Find out about the organisations in your area that offer advice and support for those people who suffer from *one* of the non-sensory conditions described in this chapter. If services are not provided in your area, how can people with this condition get help and support?

Learning difficulties

Into this category fall people with an IQ of less then 70, and they will have a history of delayed development and slow acquisition of living skills.

There are different degrees of severity resulting in varying levels of disability. The usual classifications include:

- moderate learning difficulties;
- severe learning difficulties;
- Down's syndrome;
- phenylketonuria;
- behavioural problems.

About 2 per cent of the UK population can be described as having one of these conditions. Some, such as Down's syndrome and phenylketonuria, are congenital or inherited conditions, others appear to be due to damage before or at birth, while about 15 per cent have no known cause.

Moderate and severe learning difficulties

People with moderate learning difficulties can lead independent lives if therapy and training are provided throughout their childhood and early adult lives.

Those with severe learning difficulties may need life-long care and protection.

Down's syndrome

People suffering from Down's syndrome (caused by an extra chromosome) have a typical facial characteristic of a broad, flat face with slant eyes. They will have developmental problems, which may be complicated with heart defects. They may have moderate to severe learning difficulties. There is no cure and treatment involves training as for others with learning difficulties.

Phenyl-ketonuria

Phenylketonuria is a condition in which individuals are unable to use a protein called phenalynin, which builds up in the brain causing damage, and if not treated can result in severe learning difficulties. The condition can be diagnosed soon after birth by the routine use of a blood test called the Guthrie test. If the child is found to have the condition then a diet with no or little phenalynin is given and normal development should follow.

Behavioural problems

This condition includes people displaying poor or maladjusted behaviour, and can occur at any time in life. In children and adolescents it may be displayed as obsessive, disruptive or solitary behaviour. In adults it may show itself as anxiety or depression. It is really a failure to adjust to life or changes in life, resulting in an inability to cope with home, school, work or social activities.

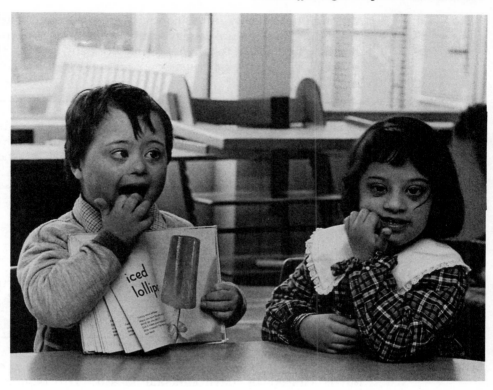

Children suffering from Down's syndrome may have special learning needs.

Treatment may include child or family guidance, psychotherapy or specialist residential care. In most cases it is temporary and disappears if the cause is removed or if the individual is helped to adjust. Some young people may grow up to be severely maladjusted if treatment is not successful.

Mental illness

There are two categories of mental illness:

- *psychoses* – schizophrenia, manic depression;
- *neuroses* – depression and anxiety, including phobias.

Psychoses

The psychoses are severe disorders in which the individual loses touch with reality and often does not realise that they are ill. They view life in a distorted way, often having hallucinations, delusions, thought disorders, emotional disturbances, mania and depression.

The exact cause or causes are not known, but it is thought that they are due to a disorder of the brain function.

Treatment by drugs can be effective in controlling symptoms. Some victims can lead fairly normal lives, but with others their social and emotional development is affected in such a way that they need long-term care.

Neurosis

Neurosis describes a range of symptoms of psychiatric disorders in which the sufferers remain in touch with reality and often know they are ill.

143

Although the severity of the condition may fluctuate, often in response to stress, the victims do not display severe behavioural abnormalities. However, they may find it hard to join in normal work and social activities. Treatment is usually by therapy or drugs or a combination of both

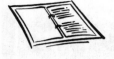

Case study

Mr and Mrs Carr have just been told that their newborn baby daughter, Maria, has been born with Down's syndrome. They have two other children, a son Jonathan (9 years) and a daughter Emma (12 years); neither of whom have had any developmental problems. Mrs Carr was intending to return to her work as a departmental store manager when the baby was three months old. Mr Carr works shift hours in the local car factory, where he has worked for the last 15 years when they moved into the area.

To do

Given the above case history decide what help and support this family is going to need. What help can each of the service providers offer? (Health, social services, education and voluntary.)

Summary

Many factors lead to people having disabilities, some genetic or inherited, others caused by environmental factors. The degree to which these disabilities affect people's lives depends upon the severity of the disability, the person's personality and the help they receive.

A disability which may cause a severe handicap for one person, may not affect another person as much, due to their individual circumstances. For example, one person who has been blinded may give up and become a recluse, expecting others to provide total care, while another in the same situation may overcome the disability by accepting special training, developing other skills and continuing to lead a normal full life.

To do

Try and think of people who have disabilities, whom you know, either personally or through the media. How have they coped? How have they overcome their disabilities? Which organisations did or could have helped them?

Key points

- Genetic and environmental factors both play a part in determining the way people develop.
- The blueprint for a person's development is carried on genes, half of which are inherited from one parent and half from the other.

- Genetics may determine the potential, but environmental factors determine whether the full potential is reached or not.
- Disabilities may be caused by genetic or environmental factors.
- Congenital disabilities are those people are born with, acquired disabilities are those which manifest due to injuries or illness after birth.
- Disabilities may be physical, psychological or a combination of both.
- Many people with disabilities can be helped to overcome the effects through treatment.
- There are many organisations in each sector of care that can offer advice, support or care for many disabilities.

9 *Human development and behaviour*

Following Chapter 8 where we discussed the factors that can affect development, in this chapter we are going to look at the way development takes place between the age of eight until death. The areas discussed are:

- physical;
- intellectual;
- emotional and social.

Physical development

After the age of seven children continue to grow and develop physically at a steady rate, although there may be growth spurts. Their physical skills develop from the base already established, with dexterity, agility and strength showing improvements as they practise and learn new tasks.

The next important landmark in this area of development is puberty, when the body becomes fully capable of reproduction.

At puberty there is a dramatic change in the growth rate, including:

- an increase in body size;
- changes in the shape and composition of the body;
- rapid development of the reproductive systems;
- development of the secondary sex characteristics.

Puberty usually occurs between the ages of 10 and 15 in both sexes, with the change taking between 1½ to 6 years in girls and from 2 to 5 years in boys. There is a great variance in both the age and duration determined by:

- inherited genes;
- setting of an internal clock;
- environmental influences.

Glands and hormones

Much of the control for the process is by the glands and hormones in the body, with the hypothalamus gland being the master. The hypothalamus is situated at the base of the brain, just above the pituitary gland. When it matures it sends messages to the pituitary gland, which is an endocrine gland releasing hormones or chemical messengers into the bloodstream. Hormones stimulate the activity of other tissues in the body.

In the case of the pituitary it releases many different hormones, and is known as the master gland because of the control it has over many body functions.

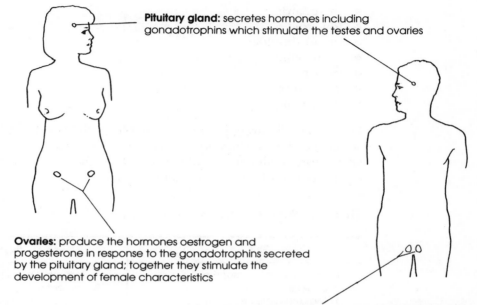

Pituitary gland: secretes hormones including gonadotrophins which stimulate the testes and ovaries

Ovaries: produce the hormones oestrogen and progesterone in response to the gonadotrophins secreted by the pituitary gland; together they stimulate the development of female characteristics

Testes: produce the hormone testosterone in response to the gonadotrophins secreted by the pituitary gland; together they stimulate sperm production and the development of other male characteristics

The pituitary glands and gonads

During puberty the pituitary is important in that it releases:

- a *growth hormone* that is essential for all the tissue growth;
- *gonadotrophic hormones*, which act specifically on the gonads or sex organs of the body.

There are two gonadotrophic hormones:

- FSH or follicle-stimulating hormone, which encourages the growth of eggs and sperm, and stimulates the production of some sex hormones;
- LH or luteinising hormone which stimulates the production of other sex hormones.

The gonads are:

- the ovaries in the female, producing eggs;
- the testes in the male, producing sperm.

They also produce the hormones that are responsible for the bodily changes of adolescence. These hormones are called *androgens* in the male, of which testosterone is the most important, and *oestrogen* in the female. It is these hormones that are responsible for the development of the secondary sex characteristics such as:

- the beard;
- low voice;
- broad shoulders;   male
- body hair;
- breasts;
- wider hips;   female
- body hair.

Development during puberty is variable, both in onset and duration, but the sequence of events tends to be the same. Hands and feet tend to reach adult size before adult height and weight are reached. The following table shows the sequence of changes for females and males.

Table 9.1   Sequential changes in maturity

Girls	Boys
1. Initial breast development	1. Testis and penis growth begins
2. Straight pubic hair	2. Straight pubic hair
3. Maximum growth	3. Early voice changes
4. Kinky pubic hair	4. First ejaculation
5. Menarche (periods begin)	5. Kinky pubic hair
6. Axillary hair	6. Maximum growth
	7. Axillary hair
	8. Marked voice changes
	9. Beard
	10. Indentation of temporal hair line

Over the last 100 years there have been changes in the ages of maturity. Today children are growing up faster, with girls now achieving adult height at 16 years rather than 19, and boys at 18 rather than 24 years. Girls are also having their first period about three years earlier than they were. Better nutrition and health are thought to be the reasons why potential is achieved earlier, but it is now thought that this situation has stabilised and the genetic influences are now the determining factor in the varying rates of development.

Mature adults

After the completion of puberty the mature adult experiences very few physical changes until middle or old age is reached. In females the next important milestone is that of the menopause, usually occurring at about 45 to 55 years. The menopause describes the pattern of changes that occur when the level of oestrogen, produced by the ovaries, is reduced. Ova in the ovaries are no longer produced, and there are increases in the amounts of other hormones. Common problems associated with the menopause are:

- hot flushes;
- loss of interest in sex;
- changes in metabolism which may later be revealed in conditions such as
  - osteoporosis (a thinning of the bones),
  - heart disease.

Many women suffer no ill effects from the menopause, and the cessation of periods, and therefore risks of pregnancy, may be welcomed. However, if symptoms are severe the modern treatment often recommended is hormone replacement therapy (HRT), which prevents many of the symptoms or lessens the effects of the menopause.

Old age

Physical and physiological changes associated with ageing usually start to occur after the age of 60, although some, such as greying hair, baldness and lack of libido, can occur well before this age. The ageing process may affect many different parts of the body, and the changes may occur singly or have a cumulative effect, with one deficiency causing another. For example, pain from arthritis may prevent a person from taking a balanced diet, because of the problems with shopping and cooking.

Some effects, such as the hair turning grey or white, or men going bald, do not physically affect people's lives, although some people may react emotionally to these signs of ageing.

To do

Discuss both the positive and negative conditions that you think develop as part of the ageing process.

Some of the common conditions that *may* occur in the ageing process are as follows.

Osteo-arthritis

This is a condition usually affecting the weight-bearing joints of the body such as:

- the hips;
- knees;
- backbone or spine.

It is thought that this condition develops through wear and tear, which affects the cartilage covering the surfaces of the bones within the joints. Genetics and diet are other factors which may influence the development of this condition.

It is a painful condition as the joints become inflamed and it can lead to changes in posture and some curving of the spine. Because of the pain

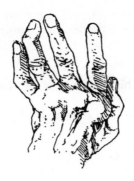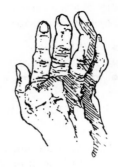

Arthritic hands

involved with movement, people tend to become less mobile and it therefore has many other effects on people's lives. As well as their physical lives osteo-arthritis can affect people both emotionally and socially. Fortunately, today much can be done to help these sufferers, including:

- treatment with drugs;
- physiotherapy;
- occupational therapy;
- surgery.

To do

Under the three headings of physical, emotional and social, list all the ways that osteo-arthritis may adversely affect a person's life.

Arteriosclerosis

This is a condition that affects the arteries of the body. As the body ages so the walls of the arteries become harder and less elastic, therefore restricting the volume of blood carried to all the body tissues. This condition can also be worsened by a condition known as atherosclerosis, when fatty deposits are laid down on the linings of the arteries, thus restricting the flow of blood even more. These conditions increase the tendency of people to have heart attacks or strokes. Strokes are either a haemorrhage or blood clot in the brain, causing damage to the brain cells.

Arteriosclerosis is one ageing condition that is affected by people's lifestyles and habits such as:

- smoking;
- high alcohol consumption;
- overeating.

Other factors are:

- high stress levels;
- lack of exercise;
- a diet high in animal fats or cholesterol.

Osteoporosis This is a condition where the bone tissue loses some of its mass, and becomes more porous and brittle, resulting in a greater tendency for bones to fracture or break. It is commonest in post-menopausal women, and the lack of the hormone oestrogen is thought to have a controlling influence over the balance of calcium in the bones and tissues. Other factors such as:

- genetics,
- lifestyle factors,
- lack of calcium,
- lack of vitamin D, and
- lack of exercise throughout life,

are all thought to be important factors.

Treatment for post-menopausal women is usually hormone replacement therapy (HRT), together with a recommendation to take more exercise.

Teeth Many elderly people in Britain lose their own teeth and rely on dentures or false teeth. It is thought that a diet high in sugar is partly responsible for the decay of teeth, so a preventive course is the restriction of sugar, particularly sweets and biscuits, and regular dental check-ups throughout life. Once dentures have been fitted it is important that these are checked at regular intervals, as it is possible for the gums to shrink and then the dentures become loose and ill-fitting, giving problems with eating and speech.

Memory The brain is made up of billions of brain cells or neurones and is responsible for all of the body's activities. After the age of about 25 years some of these brain cells die every day and are not replaced. With most functions this does not seem to have any effect, but it does seem to impair short-term memory. The result is that many older people can remember clearly events that happened in the distant past, but not what happened yesterday. Genetics seem to play an important part in the age at which this occurs, and there is no real treatment for this condition.

Dementia Dementia is a general decline in all areas of mental ability, with decreasing intellectual ability being the most obvious feature.

Alzheimer's disease About 10 per cent of dementia cases are caused by injuries or treatable illnesses, but the majority of cases are due to Alzheimer's disease. Alzheimer's is currently completely irreversible as there is a gradual loss of brain cells and shrinkage of the brain substance.

Symptoms could include:

- forgetting recent events;
- severe unpleasant personality traits;
- physical violence;
- depression;
- deterioration in personal habits, so they become dirty;

151

- incoherent speech;
- emotional outbursts;
- embarrassing behaviours.

Treatment can include sedation, but these people need a lot of personal care, either in their own homes or in residential settings. If being cared for by families, the care services will need to provide a lot of support for those providing the care.

To do

Discuss how different aspects of lifestyle may have affected the way that older people whom you know have aged.

Lifestyles

As can be seen from the above information there are many different factors involved in the process of ageing. The one that most people have control over is lifestyle, the way we live our lives. Therefore each of us can have some control over the ageing process in our own bodies. In this section we are going to look at some of these factors:

- smoking;
- diet;
- exercise.

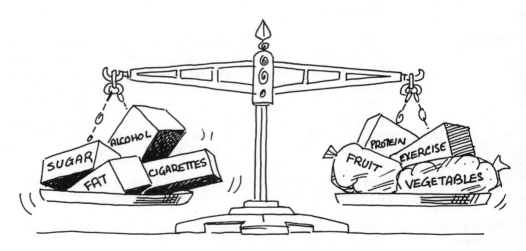

Smoking

Smoking has ageing effects, as well as contributing to the development of diseases such as:

- cancer;
- heart and lung disease;
- gastric problems.

People who smoke also tend to show ageing in the skin earlier than other comparative non-smokers.

Other side-effects cause problems, which lead on to other difficulties, for example:

- breathlessness, which can affect the willingness and capability of the person to take regular exercise;
- little interest in food so they do not always take an adequate balanced diet.

Diet

This is discussed more fully in Chapter 10, but diet is an important aspect of development. It is essential that all people have a regular, well-balanced diet containing all the essential foods, such as:

- protein,
- carbohydrates,
- roughage,
- minerals, and
- vitamins,

in the correct proportions for their needs. A lack of any of these can affect development, as can an imbalance. These days it is genarally accepted that intakes of sugars and fats should be limited, as should salt.

Exercise

All people need a certain amount of exercise in order to maintain good body functioning. Exercise helps:

- to promote healthy heart, circulatory and respiratory systems;
- to maintain good body tone and a level of fitness;
- to prevent obesity or problems of overweight;
- to prevent osteoporosis;
- to promote a sense of well-being, and stimulate alertness and a general level of interest.

To do

Develop a suitable fitness programme either for yourself or another specific individual, giving reasons for your choice.

Intellectual development

Preoperational stage

By the age of seven most children will have reached what Piaget called the preoperational stage of development, which means that the child learns to accept the conservation principles. In other words the child can accept that the amount of a substance does not change when its shape changes or if it is divided into different parts. For example, if a litre of water is poured into different shaped jugs children are aware that it is the same amount.

Concrete operational stage

Between the ages of 7 and 12 the child goes through the concrete operational stage. At this stage the child can begin to master other logical manipulations, such as sorting and ordering objects on the basis of a dimension such as

153

height or weight. This child can also draw maps of routes that they know well. Piaget called this a 'concrete operational' stage because the child can only deal with concrete objects, although they may be using abstract terms to describe them.

Formal operational stage

The formal operational stage begins at about 11 or 12, at adolescence, when children can begin to think in purely symbolic and abstract forms, and begin to solve problems. Piaget summarised this stage as:

- the ability to consider all the possibilities;
- work out the consequences for each hypothesis;
- confirm or deny these consequences.

This ability to think of possibilities beyond what is the present reality leads the adolescent to think of alternative ways of doing things and can bring them into dispute or conflict with an older age group. They often see solutions to problems in ideological ways and become very interested with metaphysical problems.

Although many people have criticised Piaget's work, most accept the existence of his sequences, but point out that there may be many more variations in the ages at which these occur. Factors that can affect the rate of development include:

- poor home situation;
- poor schooling, including poor tuition;
- absenteeism from school;
- poor relationships;
- low level of basic learning skills, e.g. reading;
- low self-esteem;
- low motivation.

Some psychologists would argue that these factors can only have so much bearing on the level of attainment, and that genetic factors are the ones that govern the ultimate potential. The nature–nurture (genetic–environment) debate has been going on for many years, with both extreme viewpoints given, i.e. final achievement is *only* to do with genetics, or is *only* to do with environmental issues. The majority of people now accept that the two interrelate. It is probable that genetics lay down the ultimate potential and that environmental factors dictate the degree to which this is realised.

To do

Think up different ways to demonstrate the three stages:

- preoperational;
- concrete operational;
- formal operational.

If possible, test them out with young people of the appropriate ages.

There are two other important aspects to cognitive development, namely field dependent and field independent, and right or left brain dominant.

Field dependent and field independent

These terms refer to the way people receive, perceive and process information. People are thought to fall into either one or the other style of thinking.

Field-independent thinkers are those who:

- perceive things discreetly;
- separate the different component of the whole.

Field-dependent thinkers:

- find it difficult to separate out the different component parts;
- are influenced by the background or context in which the item is embedded.

For example, field independents are more likely to be able to isolate the different musical instruments when listening to a piece of music. The field dependent will only hear the whole sound.

These differences can affect the way people prefer to learn and also other aspects of their lives.

- Field dependents prefer discussion and democratic styles of teaching, whereas the field-independent learner prefers formal lectures.
- Field dependents are more affected by criticism.
- Field dependents prefer social occupations, while field-independents prefer analytical occupations.
- Field dependents are more influenced by their peers and by authority.
- Field dependents are more socialised.
- Field dependents are better at remembering social information.

This type of information is important in that it may affect the person's ability, with the field independent being better at maths and sciences, and the field dependents better at the social sciences. It may also affect their career choices, with the field dependents likely to choose careers in education and caring.

To do

Classify yourself and the others you know as field dependent or field independent, giving reasons for your choice. Draw a simple bar chart to show the results.

Right or left brain dominant

The human brain is divided into two hemispheres which look alike but have very different functions. Table 9.2 illustrates some of the differences.

Table 9.2 Left and right side functions of the brain

Left	Right
Verbal	Non-verbal
Analytic	Synthetic
Symbolic	Concrete
Abstract	Analogic
Temporal	Non-temporal
Rational	Non-rational
Digital	Spatial
Logical	Intuitive
Linear	Holistic

To do

Using a dictionary or other reference book, write down definitions of the words in Table 9.2. As a group classify yourself as right or left brain dominant, and draw graphs to show the results.

One of the problems that right brain dominant people have is that, generally speaking, the education system favours left brain responses. It tends to rely on:

- sequenced,
- verbal,
- numerical,
- analytical functions,

and not use:

- non-verbal knowing,
- intuition,
- insight,

as part of the learning processes.

Adult development

All of the above factors can influence the intellectual development of a child, but does development stop when the child has gained the formal operational stage? If one thinks of childhood intelligence as mainly the acquisition of knowledge, then adult development can be thought of as how that knowledge is used. These stages can be thought of as four separate developments.

The achieving stage

In young adulthood knowledge is used to pursue careers and families. This entails using the knowledge gained in everyday problem-solving situations. Once this stage has been mastered the older adult can move on to the next stage.

156

The responsibility stage	At this stage the cognitive skills are used for social responsibility. This entails accepting responsibility for family, work situations and the community.
Executive stage	If the person is employed in a responsible situation in the workplace, the next attainment may be that of executive stage. These people will have high levels of responsibility, and will need to monitor all activities within the organisation. Not everyone will be in a position where they can progress on to this stage.
The reintegration stage	The final stage in adult development is that which occurs after retirement. Then the need to acquire new knowledge is less important and the person tends to focus more on to self, going through the reintegration stage. They are less likely to waste time on things that have no meaning for them, and they tend only to problem solve if it is an everyday problem which affects them. To summarise, adult development focuses less on the acquisition of knowledge, but more on the use of the knowledge gained and in the gaining of competence.

To do

Think of a range of people from different age groups, and classify them into the four different stages: achieving, responsibility, executive and reintegration. Give examples that provide the reasons for your categorisation.

As indicated earlier memory, especially short-term memory, can be affected by ageing, but people of all ages still have a capacity to learn. It is important that, throughout their lives, adults maintain an interest in things around them and continue to tackle new problems involving the cognitive or intellectual processes. Many older people, when asked what has kept them young, have answered by indicating that they have maintained or found new interests throughout their lives, that every day they have learned something new or discovered a different aspect to everyday things. Like all other parts of the body the intellectual aspects need to be regularly exercised in order to keep fit.

Emotional and social

Through adolescence into adulthood and throughout adult life there are certain aspects of development and behaviour that are very important. These include:

- identity;
- relationships;
- work;
- morality.

Perhaps the link running through all of these aspects is personality.

157

Personality development

Personality can be defined as the sum of a person's traits, habits and experiences. Although there are many schools of thought about what precisely personality is most people agree that it is made up of four component parts:

- *temperament* – the nature of a person's responses;
- *intelligence* – capabilities;
- *emotion* – feelings, attachments;
- *motivation* – moral standards, aspirations.

The way a person's personality develops is a result of the interaction between genetic and environmental factors. Therefore, although each baby shows aspects of an individual personality at birth, that personality continues to develop throughout life as a result of the other aspects of development and the experiences gained throughout life.

Two important aspects of personality are:

- *self-concept* – the way people see themselves;
- *self-esteem* – the way they value themselves.

Obviously the two factors are closely related, for if people see themselves as having many positive characteristics, then they probably also value themselves in a positive manner. In order for people to develop this positive way of looking at themselves it is important that others value them and value the things that they achieve. The role of their families, peer groups, teachers, employers and society at large all have a part to play in this development.

If individuals are shown to be viewed negatively or as worthless then they will see themselves in this light. Society often puts values on certain achievements, such as:

- the passing of examinations;
- the way people look;
- jobs;
- wealth;
- sporting achievements;
- social achievements, including their success within relationships.

If an individual 'fails' in any of these areas then the self-image takes a beating and the person views themselves less positively. If people view themselves in a negative way then they may become:

- depressed;
- unable to cope; or
- rebellious and turn to crime or deviant behaviour.

In some societies whole groups of people can be affected by the way they feel they are perceived by others. This happens when groups of people are stereotyped, or labelled, by characteristics that are viewed as negative or worthless by the rest of society. One such example in current British society is those who are unemployed.

To do

Discuss within the group all the environmental factors that have affected your own self-concept and self-esteem. Which are the most positive and negative factors? Which have affected you most? List groups in Britain that are viewed either by themselves or by others as having a poor or negative self-image. Why do you think this has happened?

An important aspect of personality development in the adolescent is that of establishing an identity. Identity means having a realistic self-concept, including recognition within society. This process goes through many stages including:

- *physical* – the acceptance of the body and its capabilities;
- *sexual* – the acceptance of the female and male roles, and the role that sexuality will play in people's lives;
- *social* – the acceptance of their role within groups and society;
- *vocational* – the acceptance of the type of work and interests that they enjoy and in which they can achieve;
- *moral* – relates to the belief and value systems;
- *ideological* – holding very strong views about the world and how it is run, in that things are seen in terms of 'simple', generalised solutions and with little patience for the explanations of their elders, bringing conflict with others;
- *psychological* – which incorporates all the other stages when people can be happy with their own individual identity.

Adolescents eventually become young adults, but when does this occur? In Britain the legal age of adulthood is 18 years, but has the individual really achieved adulthood then? Adulthood is marked by a number of factors including:

- leaving school and getting a job;
- getting married;
- becoming a parent;
- leaving home and moving to a new place of residence.

The timing and order of these factors can be very varied, but society can frown upon differences in the ordering of some of these factors. For example, some societies expect adults to be economically independent before they get married and set up their own homes; or they expect people to get married before they become parents. Different societies view these factors in different ways.

Relationships

Part of development is the evolvement of different relationships. Children go through many different stages, but until early adolescence most older children form friendship groups with children of the same sex, sharing the same range of interests. Within their families they usually accept the authority

159

of their parents, and in society they generally accept the authority of the adult. As they get older they are more likely to challenge this automatic authority as they establish their own identity.

The adolescent, as part of their development, becomes increasingly aware of their sexual development and the development of their sexuality. Sexual attitudes are learned in a complex way including:

- the attitudes in the home and their peer group;
- the timing of entry into sexual behaviour;
- the choice of reference groups in the making of sexual decisions.

Many parents find it embarrassing to discuss sexual behaviour with their children. This negative response is often perceived by the young person as meaning that sex is 'dirty' and has guilt feelings associated with it. Parental messages can be conveyed both verbally and non-verbally, both being very important, but the latter probably being the most subtle. If the child feels that sex is something not to be discussed, then the subject becomes secret and has negative feelings attached to it.

These negative feelings can then conflict with messages the child picks up from the media which often extol the positive aspects of sex through pop songs and through portrayals on television. Peer group attitudes can also be conflicting and the adolescent often resolves these conflicts through sexual humour. However, most young people go through the same stages in the formation of sexual relationships and sexual decision making.

The first move from the child playing with groups of the same sex is to form mixed groups in large numbers, such as youth clubs, which then develops into forming small groups, double dating and finally single dating.

Running with these stages are the first experiments or discovering of hetero-sexual experiences (but see below for a discussion on homosexuality). The sequence is normally:

- embracing;
- kissing;
- light caressing;
- petting;
- heavy petting;
- intercourse.

The ages at which these stages are enacted are influenced by many factors, including the conflicting messages already discussed. However, much research shows that peer group pressure is probably the most influential, together with the reluctance to appear unsophisticated. In the British culture it is usually the female who controls the decision making and is the partner who determines the stage of sexual behaviour that she will allow.

Choosing a partner

It is still the norm in this society that most adults will form a monogamous relationship with a partner from the opposite sex. Many of these monogamous partners will get married.

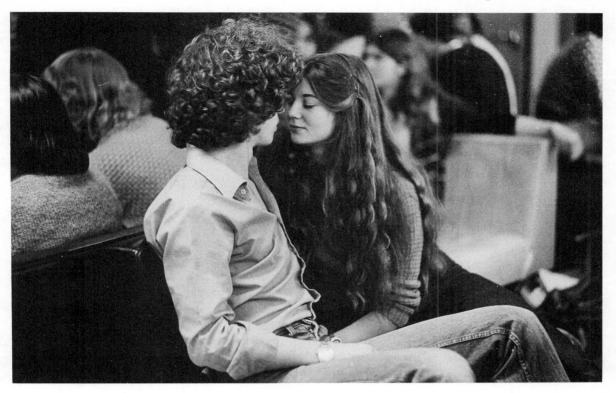

What factors influence the choice of partner? The most common reasons given are:

- falling in love;
- legitimization of sexual relationship;
- satisfying needs of companionship and sharing;
- providing security and legal rights for children;
- conformity and social expectations.

The average ages for marriage are 24 for a man and 22 for a woman, with over 90 per cent of the British population marrying before the age of 35.

What is meant by falling in love? Much time has been devoted to this question, with the consensus being that there are different factors involved including:

- *emotionally* – the feelings of companionship and caring;
- *passion* – arousal and physiological desire;
- *exclusivity* – the special relationship that excludes all others.

In other words, it includes aspects of intimacy, passion and caring.

While marriage or a monogamous heterosexual relationship is the norm in our society, it must be accepted that for some individuals this is not the desired state. Homosexuality, the establishing of a relationship with

161

someone of the same sex, is now much more readily acceptable. The reasons why some people prefer these relationships has not been established, but some people still perceive these relationships to be abnormal.

Lifelong marriages or relationships are not always the norm, with about one in three marriages ending in separation and divorce. However, many divorced people marry for the second or even third time.

To do

Discuss the reasons why you think separation and divorce have become much more widespread. What effects do you think this increase has on society as a whole?

As well as a partnership with another person the adult will usually have many other forms of relationships throughout life. These include:

- parenthood;
- working relationships;
- friendships.

Parenthood

Parenthood can occur at any stage after puberty and in a woman the ability to have children ceases with the menopause. In men the ability to father a child can extend well into old age, although fertility does decrease.

With the introduction of contraception, and the fact that these days contraception is readily available and can be very reliable, parenthood should be a form of relationship that is entered into with deliberation. However, there are still many pregnancies that occur without planning, and some women may continue with the pregnancies, but for others termination or abortion is the solution.

To do

Find out about the different forms of contraception, list their reliabilities, and the pros and cons for each type. Sources for this information include health education or promotion units, family planning clinics and doctors' surgeries.

Parenthood brings with it many responsibilities, and legally the parents are responsible for their children until they reach the age of 18. Many young parents do not realise the pressures that raising a family can put on their own relationship or the financial implications of raising a child.

In today's society these pressures can be increased by the increasing isolation of the parents. Many family groups are now limited to a nuclear family, just the parents and their children, whereas two generations ago most families were extended, with the grandparents and aunts and uncles living locally, and able to offer help and support. Added to these pressures are economic or financial matters, with many young couples needing to have two wages coming into the household in order to meet their financial commitments. Taking all these factors into account, it is most important that parenthood is planned for and that the prospective parents have some real understanding of the life commitment they are making when deciding to become parents.

Some people may make a decision not to have children, but very often there are many social pressures applied to them. Relatives, friends or society generally can imply that not having a family is abnormal, and that it is *normal* to produce a family. Some couples may wish to have a family, but are unable to, due either to some physical or psychological reason. Sometimes they can be helped by treatment or they may look for a solution by adopting or fostering a child or children.

To do

What are the issues that you think should be discussed before a couple decide to become parents? Draw up a table of pros and cons, then discuss your table with the others. If there are differences of opinion, why do you think this has occurred?

To summarise, these days people have a choice about becoming parents and ideally this should be an informed decision. For some, having children will be desirable, for others their choice is to be childless and they should not be pressured into changing their minds. Perhaps couples should have their discussions and make their decisions before entering into a long-term partnership as differences between the couple on this subject may well destroy the relationship.

Work and other relationships

For many the working environment provides a source for satisfying non-sexual relationships. The companionship of people with the same working interests can provide the feelings of belonging and worth that are essential to all. However, work can also cause many areas of conflict. It is important that people have an element of choice in the type of work that they do, but it is equally important for them to enjoy their work. Sometimes people are promoted or placed in positions in which they find their role difficult and then this can cause a great deal of stress.

There are many different types of management style, and both managers and the managed will find some styles easier than others to work with. Some senior managers can find the loneliness and the responsibilities of their position very stressful and may affect their health. Stress at work can result in many illnesses including:

- depression;
- heart problems;
- high blood pressure;
- ulcers.

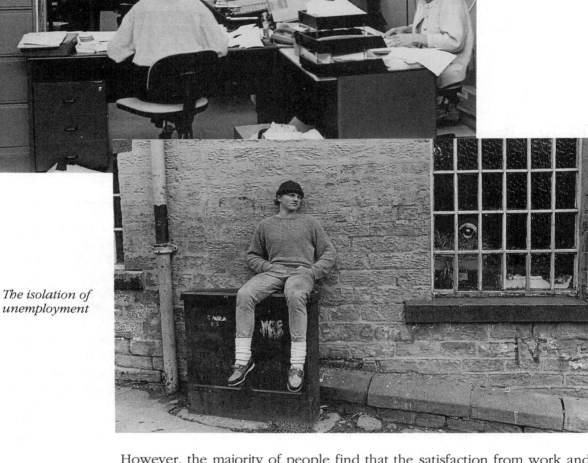

The isolation of unemployment

However, the majority of people find that the satisfaction from work and the relationships at work bring pleasure and fulfilment. One of the things that work does provide is a sense of being somebody, indeed the question that is first asked when meeting somebody new is 'What do you do for a living?' For people who are unemployed the fact that they have no job often means that they:

- have no sense of identity or sense of worth;
- can be deprived of friendship and companionship from other workers (in places of high unemployment it is often found that unemployed people will form their own social groups);

- can be isolated;
- have a reduced income and therefore the inability to join some other social activities.

Taking all these factors into account it is possible to begin to understand the difficulties that can face the long-term unemployed.

Social friendship and social groupings are also formed by adults, sometimes as couples, but also sometimes as individuals. These friendships may be purely social when people get together purely to enjoy each other's company, but they may also be based on common interests, such as clubs or societies. In some cases business is linked to pleasure and it is often said of British business that many decisions are made over lunch or on the golf course! Some social clubs will be favoured by a single sex, while others will normally have a very mixed membership.

To do As a group discuss the different types of adult relationships you have. What clubs or organisations exist in your locality? Try and organise both your relationships and the organisations under general headings, and decide what functions each type of relationship or organisation fulfils.

Development of morality

In a society without choice there is no reason for decision making, but in most societies there are choices and people have to make decisions. These judgements are often based on a personal philosophy, but how does this philosophy originate, and how do people learn 'right from wrong'?

The whole process is an interaction of many different processes and factors. Children are not born moral or immoral, but these characteristics develop as a result of interaction with the environment. An individual's innate drives may play some part, but other factors are likely to be more important.

Aspects of environmental factors are those of:

- modelling;
- imitation;
- reinforcing.

Children and young people will copy others who have influence with them, or whom they admire, such as:

- parents;
- teachers;
- popular heroes such as sports personalities, filmstars or pop singers.

If a person's behaviour is rewarded in a way that is desired by that individual, then the behaviour is likely to be repeated.

165

Young people also develop a social perspective that allows them to be aware of the effects that their behaviour has on others and of the consequences of their own behaviour. Their developing cognitive skills also enable them to process morally relevant information and to make informed decisions.

The result of these interactions of parental values and behaviours, experiences and general aspects of development is the moral development of that individual.

Each society will have its own set of rules by which it expects individuals within that society to conform. In modern society this consists of laws and social rules. Many of them are introduced to protect the vulnerable, but as society develops and changes there is a need for the rules to be amended. These amendments are often made as a result of pressure from a general shift in moral opinion. For example, when an influential part of society felt that it was immoral to make children under 14 work, laws were introduced to make it illegal.

To do

Think of as many changes to laws or social rules that have arisen from a change in moral attitudes. What laws or rules do you think are immoral in modern society? Why? How would you change them?

There are different stages of moral development, and psychologists give different names to these stages, but the basic stages are as follows:

- 'I'll do it to avoid punishment.'
- 'I'll do it if you do something for me.'
- 'I'll do it to be nice and to have you like me.'
- 'I'll do it because it's the law.'
- 'I'll do it because we've agreed it's best for everyone.'
- 'I'll do it because it's universally right.'

These last two stages can sometimes bring people into conflict with the law, if they feel as an individual that the law itself is immoral and not fair. Responsible people who reach these stages of development can be strong campaigners for changes in the law. To summarise, the individual will be born with innate drives, which together with many environmental factors will build into a system of moral values, by which that individual will be governed in all decision making throughout life.

Summary

Although the early years of life see the quickest and most dramatic changes in all aspects of human development, the later years still see changes and developments occurring, albeit at perhaps a slower rate. Puberty is a very important milestone in physical development, the other major change in women being the menopause. Intellectual, emotional and social developments are very closely related to environmental factors, but people continue to develop and change throughout their lives.

Key points

- Puberty may occur any time between the ages of 10 to 15 years.
- Developments during puberty are controlled by hormones.
- Physical developments are achieved at earlier ages, thought to be because of better nutrition and health.
- Many older people live normal, active lives, but some physiological changes do occur, which can cause some diminishing faculties, e.g. mobility.
- It is important that adults continue to exercise both their minds and bodies in order to keep fit and active.
- Intellectual development focuses on how knowledge gained can be used.
- Self-esteem and self-perception form the basis of personality development.
- Relationships may be sexual, parenthood, friendship or working, and the nature of relationships change as people mature and age.
- Moral development, based both on inherited and environmental factors, forms the base on which adult decisions are made.

10 *Maintaining personal care*

As you will have discovered by reading through the other chapters in this book, there are many different factors responsible for moulding individuals, and for providing services for individuals; but throughout all aspects of care one principle is foremost. That principle is that each person is an individual, and that each person should be treated as an individual, with carers recognising this individuality, and providing the correct amount of care and support in order that the individual can lead the lifestyle they would choose, given their individual limitations.

All people, of all ages and both sexes, well or sick, with or without disabilities, have the same basic needs in life. The only thing that differs may be the way in which these needs are met. There are many different ways of classifying these needs, but one of the most straightforward is to think of them under two main headings:

- psychological;
- physical.

Psychological needs can be further subdivided into:

- intellectual;
- emotional;
- social.

Physical needs are those that we have for our physical well-being, e.g. food, warmth.

Intellectual needs are those that are met through learning, reading, challenges etc.

An example of an *emotional* need is the need for love and affection.

The need for friends and companions is one of the *social* needs.

To do

Under these four headings (physical, intellectual, emotional and social), think of all the needs you as an individual have? Compare your lists with others, do they vary very much?

In order to meet these needs people develop drives. These are the forces that motivate us to initiate or start behaviours in order that the need may be met. For example, if a person feels hungry they will need food. This hunger drive will initiate behaviour that will enable them to meet this need – in ancient times to go hunting, now perhaps to look in the fridge!

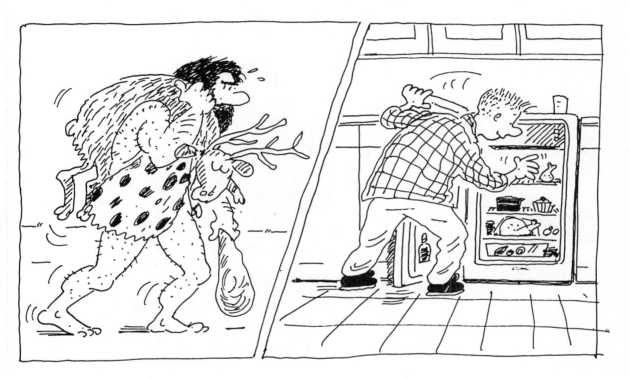

Like hunger many of the drives that people have are controlled by physiological mechanisms, others being:

- thirst;
- avoidance of pain;
- protection from the elements;
- sex.

The psychological needs that people have create different types of behaviour which are called *motives*. The behaviours that result either from drives or motives tend to be influenced by learning and the type of society in which the individual lives. For example, a person deprived of food, say a youngster in a drought-ridden country, would be driven by hunger to steal some corn, but a well-fed person from the UK who stole a bar of chocolate would be driven by some motivation other than hunger.

Abraham Maslow, a psychologist, proposed a method of classifying motives, by drawing up a hierarchy of needs. The lower level needs have to be met before the next level becomes the determinant or motivator of behaviour.

169

The base level consists of the physiological or biological needs that we are all born with, and when these are satisfied the next level of needs becomes the driver or motivator. Therefore, in societies where people are still struggling for food, shelter and safety, these are the needs determining their behaviour.

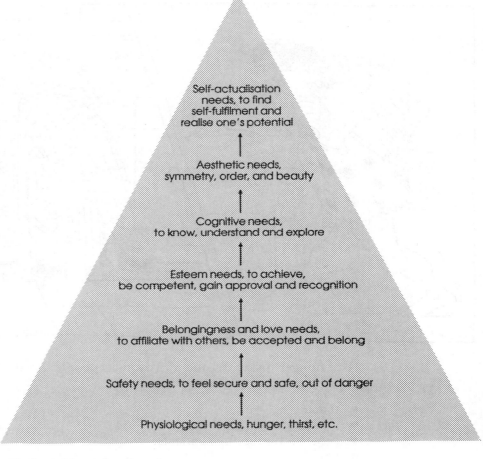

Maslow's hierarchy of needs

If you refer back to Chapter 3 you will see that the list of principles for the rights of individuals reflect this hierarchy of needs, above the base levels.

In this chapter we are going to examine the ways in which some of these basic and higher needs can be met, and where applicable mention will be made of special points for the different client groups mentioned in Chapter 1. The sections will include:

- diet;
- infection;

- cleanliness;
- managing continence;
- independence, including mobilisation and safety;
- recreation;
- coping with death and bereavement.

To do

Check who the different client groups are from Chapter 1, and using your list of needs as a guide, list some of the difficulties people from the different groups may have in meeting their own needs. How can carers help meet these needs? (Use your experiences from the workplace to help you.)

Diet

In some parts of the world there are problems in ensuring that the population has an adequate food and drink supply, with protein malnutrition being one of the main health problems in developing countries. However, within the UK there are no food shortages, but there are still problems caused by diet and food. There is a national nutritional policy to ensure that certain conditions are met, these include:

- all essential foodstuffs available to the whole population at reasonable cost;
- priority foods provided for certain sections of the community, for example free school meals for children whose families are in need, subsidised meals on wheels or lunch clubs for the elderly;
- many foods are fortified to guarantee adequate supplies of vitamins;
- foodstuffs must be free from disease;
- milk and water supplies must be free from disease;
- food handlers must be trained to a high standard of food hygiene.

Some of these measures can help to ensure that people in the UK have a safe supply of food, but it is up to individuals or their families to ensure that the diet is adequate. This means that the diet contains the right foods in the right amounts in order that the individual needs are met. This is usually called a *balanced diet*, but it will not be the same for everyone, as different people will have different needs. What are the foods required in a balanced diet, and what are the different needs?

A balanced diet

This should contain:

- sufficient calories;
- protein, fat and carbohydrate in roughly the proportions 1:1:3;
- vitamins and minerals;
- roughage or fibre;
- water.

Calories

Calories provide the energy source for the body, and a calorie is defined as: 'the amount of heat required to raise 1 litre of water 1 degree Centigrade'.

In dietary terms calories are the energy content of food; if calorie/energy content of a diet equals energy used then a steady weight is maintained.

Each person will have their daily requirement of calories, which will be dependent on their lifestyle and occupation. The more active a person is the greater their calorie requirement will be. A rough guide to daily calorie requirements is:

CALORIES

- at rest   1400–1550
- light work   2000–2750
- heavy work   3000
- during pregnancy   2500
- during lactation   3000

Calories can be found in carbohydrates, fat and protein, their average calorific values being:

- 1 g of carbohydrate   = 4 calories
- 1 g of protein   = 4 calories
- 1 g of fat   = 9 calories

Therefore, if we think of the proportions suggested for these different foods, a well-balanced diet for an average man should be made up like this:

CALORIES

- protein   70–100 g   (300–400)
- fat   70–100 g   (600–900)
- carbohydrate   500 g   (2000)

              Total   (3000–3500)

So where are these different foods found, and what other functions do they have as well as providing calories?

Proteins

Source:

- meat;
- eggs;
- milk and dairy products;
- fish;
- wheat;
- legumes – beans, peas.

Animal sources contain all the essential amino acids required by humans, whereas each vegetable source only contains some, but if a varied diet of vegetable proteins is eaten all the essential amino acids can be obtained.

Proteins are necessary for growth and tissue replacement, with the average adult requiring about 70 g a day minimum. Children use about a third of their protein intake for growth, and other groups such as pregnant women and sick people need a good supply of daily protein.

Protein cannot be stored in the body, so a daily intake should be eaten.

Fats

Source:

- eggs;
- milk and dairy products;
- fatty meats;
- oily fish – herring, salmon, trout;
- seeds – olives, sunflower.

Fats are a concentrated form of energy and a vehicle for fat-soluble vitamins.

Fats can be stored in the body and form the main reserve of energy. Today, animal fats which contain saturated fats are thought to be less healthy, and to contribute towards heart disease, so people are encouraged to take more of their supply of fats from fish or vegetable sources. In fact, recent research indicates that fish oils may help to prevent heart disease.

Carbohydrates

Sources of carbohydrates are cereals, flour, potatoes and sugars.

Carbohydrates are an energy source that is quickly available, but can be stored as glycogen in the liver and muscles in the body. These stores can also be quickly converted back into glucose, the form of carbohydrate that the body requires for energy. Carbohydrate foods are usually fairly cheap and available, but in modern society people are advised to eat carbohydrates that provide other benefits as well, rather than those, like sweets and biscuits, which basically just provide carbohydrate.

Fibre or roughage

Fibre is the cellulose element in vegetable foods, which is not absorbed. It is especially found in skins, bran and whole cereals.

Fibre provides bulk for a healthy large intestine. It provides chemicals which are useful for fat metabolism, limiting the chances of heart disease.

Mineral salts

Name	Source	Use
Calcium	Milk, cheese, fruit, vegetables	Bones, clotting of blood, muscular contractions
Phosphorous	Most foods except butter and sugar	Bones and fat metabolism
Iron	Eggs, liver, whole grains, leaf vegetables	Helps to form haemoglobin of the blood
Iodine	Fish, milk, leaf vegetables	Helps functioning of the thyroid gland

There are also many other trace elements such as potassium, copper, manganese, zinc and fluorine that are required in minute amounts to help with various body functions, most of which are found in a 'normal' diet.

Vitamins

Name	Source	Deficiency causes
A	Animal fats, as carotene in vegetables	Night blindness, and opacity of cornea – blindness
D	Fish oils and sunlight	Rickets and osteomalacia or softening of the bones
K	Leaf vegetables	Bleeding, lack of clotting
B1	Wholegrain cereals	Beri-beri, neuritis
B2	Milk, eggs, liver, kidney	Dermatitis, sore tongue
B12	Wholegrain cereals	Pernicious anaemia
Nicotinic Acid	Wholegrain cereals excluding maize	Pellagra
C	Green vegetables, fresh fruit	Scurvy, bleeding in mucous membranes

NB Neither human nor animal milk contains Vitamin C, therefore all babies need Vitamin C additives

Diets of different groups

Some people prefer one type of diet for one reason or another, but the main reasons for choosing diet restrictions are religious or philosophical.

Hindu

Many Hindus are vegetarian, not eating meat, eggs, fish or products made from them. The cow is a sacred animal, therefore the eating of beef is strictly forbidden, even by non-vegetarians. Alcohol is also strictly forbidden.

Fasting may also form part of the Hindu lifestyle, but can take different forms, usually involving restrictions rather than total fasting.

Sikh

Sikhism began in the 16th century as an offshoot of Hinduism, and many of the dietary restrictions are the same. Many Sikhs, particularly women, are vegetarian. Few eat beef, as the cow is sacred, and conservative Sikhs disapprove of alcohol.

Muslim

Dietary restrictions are laid down in the Holy Koran. No pork or pork products can be eaten, but providing that other meats are halal, they can be eaten. Halal means that the name of Allah is pronounced over the animal which is then killed as prescribed by Muslim law. Alcohol is prohibited.

Adult Muslims must fast during the 30 days of Ramadan, which means eating and drinking nothing between dawn and sunset. Some people are exempt, including elderly and infirm people, pregnant or breast-feeding women, ill people or those on a journey. Except for elderly and infirm people, the others are expected to make up the number of fasting days as soon as possible after Ramadan.

Jewish

Dietary rules or the Jewish Kashrut are followed by devout Jews. Pork or pork products, or shellfish may not be eaten. Other meats and fish can be eaten, provided they are killed by proper or kosher methods. Milk and meat must not be used together, and separate utensils must be used for cooking and eating.

Fasting takes place on Yom Kippur (the Day of Atonement), and no yeast products are allowed during the Passover or Pesach.

Rastafarian

The Rastafarian faith encourages vegetarianism, but some followers eat meat other than pork. The faith discourages the eating of processed foods that contain additives and preservatives.

Seventh-day Adventists

Seventh-day Adventists do not eat pork or pork products.

Philosophical

Some people feel that it is wrong to eat animal or animal products, as they do not feel that animals should suffer for the sake of humans. There are two main groups of diets, but there are many variations.

Vegetarians do not eat meat or meat products. Dairy products and eggs are consumed, and many vegetarians will eat fish.

Vegans will not eat meat or fish, or any fish or meat products. Therefore, vegans will only eat vegetables, fruits and products made from these.

Summary

It is important that all carers respect people's dietary preferences, and it is possible for all groups to have a balanced diet, but more care may have to be taken with clients from some groups such as vegans, who must ensure that they eat a range of protein foods that include all the amino acids, but also that they receive sufficient fat-soluble vitamins in their diet.

To do

You are a care assistant in a residential home for elderly people. The officer in charge has just asked you to help the cook prepare the menu. At least one of the residents follows a special diet of a religious group. Choose a variety of meals for the week providing all the residents with a balanced diet. Indicate how the basic requirements are being met.

As well as the food we eat it is important to store and prepare food correctly and we will discuss this topic in the next section.

Infection

Many diseases are called infections and are caused by organisms called germs. Germs which cause diseases are called pathogenic micro-organisms and are divided into two main groups, *bacteria* and *viruses*.

Bacteria are divided into groups depending on their shape, the main ones being:

- cocci (round), e.g. streptococci and staphylococci;
- bacilli (rods), e.g. tetanus bacilli and tubercle bacilli;
- vibrios (curved), e.g. cholera.

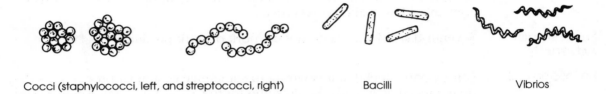

Cocci (staphylococci, left, and streptococci, right)   Bacilli   Vibrios

Viruses are very small germs that can only be seen by the use of an electron microscope, which is much more powerful than an ordinary one. Viruses cause illnesses such as colds, influenza (flu), measles and chickenpox.

Micro-organisms are not always harmful, in fact some are very useful. These harmless ones are called non-pathogenic and include those that turn milk into cheese, and those that help to break down waste organic matter such as faeces and urine.

However, many of the harmful bacteria or viruses are all around us in the everyday environment and are carried into the body by different routes:

- *inhalation* – breathed in through the mouth or nose;
- *ingestion* – swallowed usually through food or drink;
- *inoculation* – through the skin, usually via a damaged area or wound.

Some organisms can only cause one specific disease, for example the measles virus only causes measles. Others such as the streptococcus can cause tonsillitis if it lodges in the tonsils, but will cause a wound infection if it gets into an open wound.

Needs of organisms

In order to be able to prevent the spread of infection it is important to understand a little more about micro-organisms. They usually multiply very quickly, by dividing into two, about every 20 minutes or so. This means that, given the favourable conditions of warmth, moisture and food, one or two germs can become millions in a matter of days.

Not all micro-organisms need oxygen in order to live. Some organisms are very tough and can survive extremes of temperature, dryness or lack of food, by forming a tough outer covering. This is called *spore formation*. When conditions become more favourable they resume their previous lifestyle.

Given this information it makes it possible to understand which places are more likely to attract organisms and the measures that can be taken to prevent their spread.

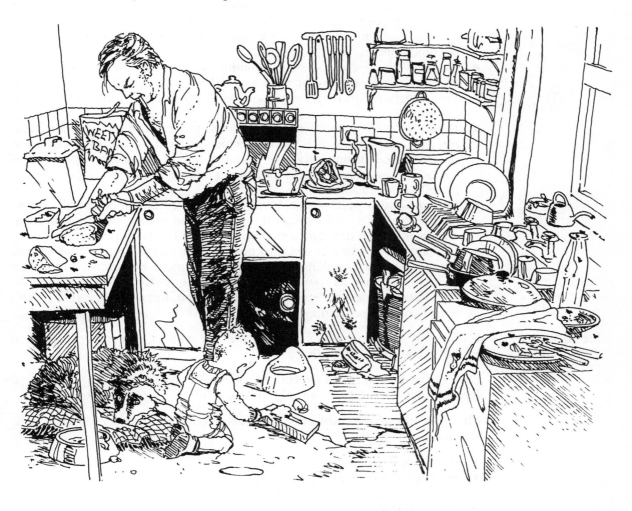

To do

Study the picture above and list all the danger points with regard to the spread of infections. How could these be prevented?

Spread of infection

Infections can be spread in many ways, and below are listed some of the most common methods.

- *Droplet infection* – whenever anyone speaks small droplets of moisture are sprayed out into the air. Any micro-organisms present in the mouth, throat or nose may be carried on the drops of moisture and breathed in by other people close to them. If someone sneezes or coughs these drops of moisture can be carried several metres and could affect most people in the same room. Colds and influenza are spread this way.
- *Direct touch* – kissing can transfer germs from mouth to mouth, and glandular fever is thought to be spread by this method. Sexual contact spreads sexually transmitted diseases. Touch can spread organisms on the skin, which can also lead to indirect infection where other things become contaminated, e.g. food.
- *Hands* – these can become contaminated by handling any infected objects or if the skin becomes damaged this wound may become infected. This infection can then be passed on in anything else that is touched, e.g. food.
- *Food and drink* – these may be infected at source, e.g. a chicken meal carrying salmonella. It is also possible for food and drink to become contaminated during processing and handling by infected people, so spreading infections. Food poisoning and typhoid are examples of infections spread this way.
- *Flies and other pests* – flies, cockroaches, mice and rats can all spread diseases, usually by feeding off contaminated objects and then passing on this infection through contaminated food eaten by people.
- *Carriers* – this name is given to people who carry diseases and spread them to others. The danger is that many of them are unaware that they carry the disease as they may not be ill themselves. Diseases that are commonly carried are streptococci and staphylococci in the throat, and typhoid or other organisms in the bowel.

Prevention of infection

Fortunately, there are many ways to prevent either the spread of infection or the infection developing.

One of the best ways to prevent the spread of infection is good personal hygiene, which will be dealt with below when we look at cleanliness.

There are also many public health measures that are undertaken in the UK, including:

- supply of clean water;
- removal and treatment of sewage;
- collection and disposal of rubbish;
- drainage systems;
- notification of infectious diseases;
- food regulations.

These measures are administered by environmental health officers who work for local authorities.

People also have some in-built defences against infection such as:

- an intact skin, which forms a good barrier;
- the acid in the stomach which kills many organisms;
- white blood cells which overcome pathogenic organisms.

Other means can be used, such as immunisation programmes, which enable the body to develop antibodies to neutralise specific organisms. However, a good level of general health is probably the best defence against infections.

To do

Find out for which infections an immunisation is available. When are these given and are there any specific groups that either receive the vaccinations or should not receive them?

Barrier nursing

If someone has an infection like gastro-enteritis (diarrhoea and vomiting), it may be necessary to isolate that person from others and to use preventive measures to stop it spreading to other people.

- All the crockery and cutlery used by the infected person should be kept apart from that used by others, and washed and sterilised by boiling after use.
- Soiled bedding and clothing should be soaked in disinfectant before washing, and sheets should be boiled if possible.
- Any bedpans, urinals or commodes should be disinfected after use.
- Paper, dressings and other disposables should either be burnt or placed in special bags for disposal by the environmental health department.
- Anyone entering the room should put on a disposable apron and gloves. When leaving the room, the apron and gloves must be disposed of.
- Personal hygiene is very important and hands should be washed after handling anything from the room.
- After the person recovers, the room and contents should be thoroughly cleaned, and well aired before further use.

Cleanliness

Personal hygiene

The term personal hygiene is used to describe the cleanliness of the individual, and the need for this applies both to the service users and the carers. Cleanliness is very important, helping to prevent the spread of disease and making life more pleasant for everyone. There are some basic rules that apply:

- handwashing should take place after going to the toilet;
- handwashing should take place before handling food, whether in preparation of food or before eating.

Care of the skin

As mentioned above an intact healthy skin is a good barrier in the prevention of infection entering through the skin. A basic way of ensuring this is to make sure that the skin is kept clean and dry. This prevents the build-up of bacteria on the surface of the skin and prevents it from cracking, enabling infection to enter.

It is important that people's individual likes and dislikes, or customs, are respected, for example:

- some people do not use soap on their faces;
- some people prefer showers to baths;
- some people like to use a bidet after going to the toilet.

Prevention of pressure sores

For those people who are immobile it is important that care is taken to prevent sores developing which can be very difficult to heal and can easily become infected. Pressure sores occur when pressure is applied to parts of the skin, especially skin over bony parts of the body:

- ankles and heels;
- knees and hips;
- buttocks and spine;
- elbows and shoulders;
- ears.

To prevent sores from developing it is important to:

- change the position of the person every two hours;
- keep the skin clean and dry;
- keep bedding clean, dry and wrinkle free;
- ensure a good, balanced diet;
- use proper lifting techniques to avoid skin dragging or scraping on the bedclothes or bedpan.

Hair care

Keeping the hair clean and tidy is very good for morale, but again it is important that individual preferences and customs are recognised. Always check how people:

- would like their hair done;
- if they wash it with shampoo or not;
- whether they like to keep their hair covered.

If you are unsure how to do someone's hair, ask for advice or get someone from the person's family to show you.

To do

Prepare a checklist of the customs of people from different cultures with regard to personal cleanliness. Use your own experiences or reference literature if necessary.

Managing continence

Many individuals, as a result of illness or disabilities, suffer from incontinence, which means losing control over elimination. This may lead to:

- urinary incontinence;
- faecal incontinence;
- both urinary and faecal incontinence.

If possible it is better to maintain continence and this can be attempted in a number of ways:

- ensure adequate toilet facilities are within easy reach;
- take the individual to the toilet regularly;
- make sure that the individual can communicate easily with the carer;
- make sure that the carer can understand the individual;
- if drugs are being administered that increase the need to pass urine (e.g. diuretics), make sure the individual is aware of this and that facilities are provided;
- ensure privacy is provided;
- prevent infections, or treat them if present;
- give reminders to people with psychological problems;
- encourage exercise to maintain muscle tone.

If the person is incontinent, then this has to be managed in such a way that any other problems are prevented or lessened.

Helping continence

There are many steps that can be taken to help with *urinary incontinence*:

- treating the underlying problem, e.g. infections or enlarged prostate in males;
- habit retraining, adopting a pattern of particular times for using the toilet, such as before and after meals;
- regular toileting;
- physiotherapy to improve muscle tone and mobility;
- adaptations of dress to ease toiletting;
- use of drugs to improve bladder capacity;
- encouraging, not limiting, fluid intake.

If the individual cannot be helped to regain continence then it is important that they retain their dignity and safeguard their skin. This can be done by:

- using protective pads and pants, such as those made by Kanga;
- use of sheath devices (light, flexible tubes that fit over the penis and drain into a bag) for men;
- indwelling catheters (fine tubes, inserted into the urethra, to enable the urine to be drained into a bag) for men and women.

Faecal incontinence is very distressing, and the causes include many of those listed for urinary incontinence, but also:

- constipation;
- diet;
- brain or spinal damage;
- overuse of aperients (drugs given to treat constipation);
- rectal problems such as cancer.

The treatment of faecal incontinence is dictated by the cause, and includes:

- following a balanced diet and plenty of fluids to prevent constipation;
- exercise to help prevent constipation;
- stressing that aperients should only be used under medical guidance;
- treatment of rectal conditions;
- if the constipation is severe it may be necessary to give an enema or suppositories.

Service provision

If the individual is being cared for at home it may be necessary to provide some other services. It is possible for help to be given with:

- laundry services;
- provision of pads;
- provision of commode.

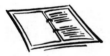

─────────────────────────── **Case study** ───────────────────────────

Mr Smith, aged 79 years, lives at home with his wife, aged 76 years. Home is a terraced, two-bedroom house, with a combined toilet and bathroom. They have always been independent, with little demand on the caring services. Recently their GP was called in when Mr Smith developed a severe bout of flu. Other than displaying all the usual signs and symptoms, both Mr and Mrs Smith were very embarrassed to admit that Mr Smith had become incontinent. Mrs Smith was finding it difficult to cope with all the extra demands.

───

To do

What help could be offered to Mr and Mrs Smith to enable them to ease their immediate problems? Which services could be called on to provide this help?

Independence ───

As we have already discussed it is important that individuals are encouraged to maintain their independence as much as possible. There are many ways in which this can be encouraged, while keeping safety in mind. There are many aids or devices on the market which, together with an adapted environment, can improve the quality of an individual's life and help towards independence.

Some of the areas in which people can be helped are:

- eating and cooking;
- dressing;
- mobility;
- leisure activities;
- home and environment.

Eating and cooking

There are many simple devices available to help with the everyday tasks of eating and cooking. Many people who have undergone neurological damage, such as strokes, may find it difficult to grip utensils, or to use one hand.

- Foam cylinders over handles of normal cutlery may help or large-handled utensils can be used.
- Combined knives and forks are available which enable people to eat with one hand.
- Shields can also be fitted to the outside of plates for the person to push the food against in order to get it on their fork or spoon.
- Many kitchen gadgets such as one-handed or electric can openers are now available.

Dressing

Many older and disabled people find buttons, laces and zips in the backs of garments very difficult to cope with. However, with a bit of thought and ingenuity there is no reason why older and disabled people cannot be smartly and fashionably dressed. Front-fastening garments, using a Velcro-type fastening, can solve a lot of problems. Elastic shoelaces can enable comfortable, safe shoes to be worn, while long-handled shoehorns help to get them on. There are also gadgets available to help with putting on socks, stocking or tights. Special incontinence pads and pants also aid independence.

Mobility

For people who are unsteady on their feet there are several supporting aids available, including:

- walking sticks;
- tripods;
- walking frames.

It is important that people are measured and the right size equipment provided. Physiotherapists can help to train people in the correct use of the equipment.

When walking is no longer possible, the individual may become a wheelchair user. There are many different types available and advice needs to be sought on an appropriate model. Unfortunately, many of the very advanced, technical models are not provided free and the individual may have to purchase it for themselves. Motorised chairs mean that it is now possible for many severely disabled people to go shopping and take part in a lot of different interests.

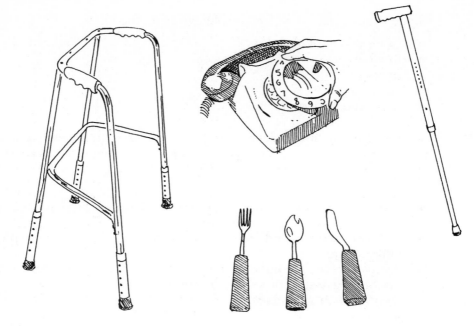

Aids for disabled people

For sports special wheelchairs have been built to enable people to take part in such activities as basketball, dancing and marathon racing.

Leisure

The idea that only young, fit people are interested in leisure activities has long been disproved. As mentioned above, many disabled people take part in sport, and there are now many clubs and events organised in many different sports. Indeed, there is an Olympic Games every four years for disabled sports people.

There is no reason why disabled people should not take part in any activity as long as properly trained supervisors and safe equipment is used. Mountaineering, sailing, skiing and parascending are all sports now available to disabled people.

However, it must be said that there is still not enough widespread sports provision for people with disabilities or access to those facilities which could be used by them.

For those preferring quieter occupations, again many clubs are available. There is an increasing demand for disabled people to join in with non-disabled people and organisations like the scouts and guides were among the first to encourage integration between able-bodied and physically disabled people. It is important for both disabled people and their carers to take part in a range of leisure activities, preferably both physical and cognitive, in order to keep both mind and body fit and active.

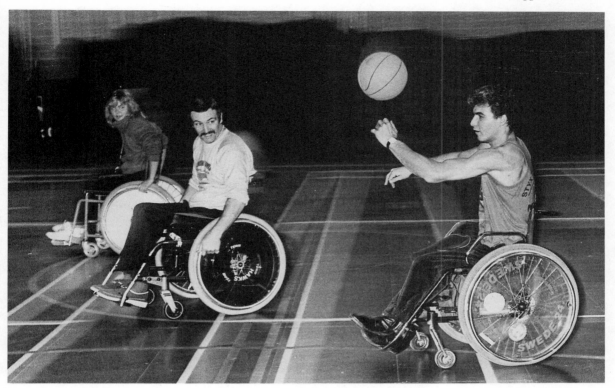

Home and environment

Modern homes do not always make the easiest environment for people with disabilities to remain independent and to have mobility in. Ways in which they can be inconvenienced include:

- narrow doorways;
- high cupboards;
- low power points;
- stairs; and
- narrow toilets and bathrooms.

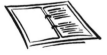

Case study

Alec McKenzie is a young man, aged 24 years. Following a car accident he suffers from paraplegia (he is paralysed from the waist down). Before his accident he was a keen basketball player, was working in a leisure centre, enjoyed going to night clubs and pubs as part of an active social life. He is shortly going to get married to Marie, the girl he was engaged to before the accident. Following his accident he was awarded compensation from his insurance company. Alec and Marie intend to use this money to build a purpose-designed bungalow for themselves.

To do

Think of the different things that could be incorporated into the design of the bungalow that will encourage independence for Alec and help him to be mobile. You may find it helpful to think about specific rooms separately.

The outside world can be a very hostile place for many people with restricted mobility. Even gardens around the house can present problems of access, not to mention maintenance!

Streets, shops, offices and public buildings are not always planned with disabled people in mind. More recently, however, much more care has been taken in the design of buildings, such as the provision of:

- ramps;
- lifts;
- wide aisles; and
- special toilet arrangements.

Despite advances, people with visual and hearing impairments can still encounter real difficulties, many of them originating from the attitudes of people.

To do

Carry out a survey of your local shopping area and indicate how easy or difficult you think it would be for people with different types of disabilities to use the facilities.

Safety

Normal rules of home safety apply when planning accommodation for people with disabilities, but it is even more important to be aware of the greater risks to the individual. Main areas of risk include:

- fire, burns and scalds;
- falling and tripping;
- cuts and wounds;
- poisoning.

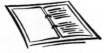

Case study

Mrs Jones is a widow, aged 76 years. She lives in a house with her unmarried, retired brother. Recently Mrs Jones started to become partially sighted through developing cataracts. She has a long history of osteo-arthritis for which she takes daily medication. She is anxious to remain in her own home while waiting for surgery on her eyes.

To do How can Mrs Jones, her brother and the caring services try to ensure that the house is a safe environment for Mrs Jones? What safeguards can be provided to protect her from accidental injury?

Recreation

This has been mentioned above with regard to those with disabilities, but it is just as important for people of all ages to include recreation and leisure activities within their lifestyles. It is important for several reasons, including:

- physical fitness;
- psychological or mental fitness;
- social involvement.

Physical fitness

Many people of all ages like to participate in sports, but this is not the only way to keep fit. Other ways include:

- walking;
- dancing;
- gardening;
- cycling.

These pursuits can either be undertaken as pure recreational activity or can be part of a normal day, such as walking or cycling to work. Physical activity helps to guard against several diseases and promotes a sense of well-being.

Psychological fitness

Keeping an interested mind is one way of staying young and maintaining an interest in life. There are many ways of using the mind in recreational activities, including:

- reading;
- crosswords or other puzzles;
- quizzes;
- orienteering;
- craft work;
- DIY;
- music, drama etc.;
- studying for interest and/or qualifications.

Social involvement

Humans are basically social beings and enjoy each other's company. It is important that as well as family and work, other social activities are included into people's lifestyles. This prevents a feeling of isolation, and can provide pleasure and stimulation. Many of the other types of recreation already mentioned involve some aspects of social behaviour.

187

To do

What recreational activities do you enjoy? Categorise them into physical, psychological, social or combined. Why do you enjoy them?

Recreation is important in order to relax, develop and keep fit. One of today's greatest causes of illness is stress, and one of the best ways of preventing stress is to relax and enjoy yourself through some form of recreation. It is something everyone can do, as it does not have to require a lot of expense – all it needs is time.

Coping with death and bereavement

This is one aspect of caring that has to be faced by all carers at one time or another. The main aspects of care in this area are:

- to allow the death to occur with dignity and as little suffering as possible,
- to recognise and respect individual customs and beliefs,
- to support family and friends, and help them through bereavement.

The dying

Carers need to provide all the physical care necessary to keep the person as comfortable and free of pain as possible.

Carers need to be:

- supportive,
- compassionate, and
- sensitive,

towards both the dying person, and their relatives and friends. Sometimes death is expected, and all of those involved may wish to prepare for it by discussing their wishes and their thoughts. Whether death is expected or sudden those involved will all go through the various stages of bereavement.

Any carers who may have been involved with the care of the dying person may also go through the process of bereavement themselves, especially if the involvement has been over a long time. These carers will need the help and support of their colleagues as they go through the stages of bereavement.

Bereavement

There are four main stages to the bereavement process:

- anticipation;
- shock;
- anger;
- acceptance.

Anticipation

Anticipation refers to the period when the dying person realises they are going to die. They may ask carers for confirmation, and these days it is

188

generally accepted that individuals have a right to know the truth about their condition. However, it is usually better if this is explained to them by an experienced person who is in a position to answer all their questions.

For relatives and friends this is the stage when they can begin to prepare for the inevitable. In the case of sudden death, this stage may be omitted and the whole of the grieving process becomes more difficult.

Shock

Both for the dying and the relatives this is a stage where disbelief and numbness take over. They don't want to believe this is happening to them. After death, the relatives may find themselves waiting for the deceased person to come home, or may hear their voice.

Anger

Again, both the dying and the bereaved go through a stage of asking 'Why me?' There is often a feeling of resentment, and the dying person may often focus this on the relatives. Carers can often be the target both from the individual and the relatives. After death the relatives often go through a period of guilt. They feel they have to blame someone and often it is themselves. Nearly everyone who has been bereaved can recall some incident where they feel they could have done something other than they did, and ask the question 'If I had done this would the person still be alive?'

Bereaved people often feel hopeless and overwhelmed by sadness at this stage.

Acceptance

When the anger fades the dying person is left with the reality of the situation and accepts the inevitability of death. This stage is often filled with a sense of peace and well-being. They are often able to offer support for their relatives at this point.

For the bereaved this is the final stage of coming to terms with their loss. They accept that the person has gone, will not be coming back and can begin to adjust to a new life. This does not mean forgetting, but accepting.

Carer's role

Carers need to understand these different stages, and the needs of both the dying and the bereaved in order to offer them the support that is needed. The time taken to go through these different stages varies from individual to individual, some going through them quickly, others taking years, and some never reaching the acceptance stage, but remaining in the anger phase.

People need to talk about:

- the death;
- the individual who has died;
- their lives together;
- how they are going to cope without them.

Unfortunately a lot of people are embarrassed by death and try to avoid the subject. This refusal can be very painful and hurtful to those recently bereaved. Expressions of sympathy can be very supportive, but also offer an opening for the bereaved to talk about their situation.

Offers of practical help are often very welcome, and the service providers should be aware of the needs and how they can fill them. Examples include:

- financial problems;
- running the home;
- coping with young children – child-care arrangements;
- mobility problems;
- loneliness.

If the statutory services cannot provide the means of filling the need, there are several voluntary organisations such as CRUSE, a national organisation with numerous local branches, who provide a specialist counselling and advice service for those who have been bereaved.

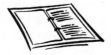

Case study

Mr Patel has just been told that he has developed secondary malignant tumours in his spine and, following discussions with the doctors, he has decided that he wants no further medical treatment other than analgesics or pain killers. His wife has said that she would like to care for him at home, and that her employers would keep her job open for her. They have four children, all in Britain, but they are married with young families of their own.

To do

How do you think this family can be helped and supported? What services may be required, both before and after Mr Patel's death? Who can provide these?

One important aspect of caring for people through dying and death must be an awareness of and respect for other's beliefs and customs. Here is a list of some of these beliefs.

Catholic — Dying person to be visited by priest and last rites said.

May be buried or cremated, no special customs.

Non-Catholic Christian — Dying person may like to be visited by clergy.

May be buried or cremated, no special customs.

Muslim — Chapter 30 of Koran to be quoted as person dies.

Body faced towards Mecca, washed by mullah or family members of the same sex.

Body dressed in white, men only attend ceremony in mosque.

Jewish — Psalms recited, Sheena is the last prayer to be said before death, at moment of death window opened to allow release of spirit.

Rabbi or holy friends carry out ritual washing of body, candles lit, someone stays with body and psalms are recited.

Body dressed in white, plain coffin, men only usually attend funeral. Body taken past house to the chapel of rest.

Hindu	Brahmin blesses the dying person, who should be at home, and on the floor. Prayers are recited in a special part of the house.
	Body is taken to the chapel of rest and cremated.
Buddhist	Supported by priest or monk, Sutra recited, meditation encouraged.
	Burial or cremation accepted.
Sikh	Scriptures are read.
	Body dressed in white.
	Cremation.
Afro-Caribbean	Immediately after death a bull roarer is swung to encourage the spirits to beckon the dead.
	Body dressed in white.
	Wake goes on for nine nights, body cremated afterwards.
Rastafarian	Prayers read.
	No special customs, but may have a nine-day wake.
Jehovah's Witness	May like to see minister.
	No special customs.
Mormon	Time for privacy and prayer twice a day for dying person.
	No special customs, burial or cremation.
Chinese	Dying person may be admitted to hospital so that spirit does not haunt house afterwards.
	Family help with laying out, body dressed in new clothes.
	Professional mourners may be employed if small family.
	Paper money burnt. Fire crackers used to frighten away spirits.
Bahai	Reciting of prayers.
	Body washed and dressed in cotton or silk shroud. Special ring placed on finger.
	Crystal, stone or firewood coffin. Body must be burned within one hour's journey of place of death. Special prayer read at internment.

191

Although this list cannot be comprehensive, it does serve to indicate that there are many different customs and practices associated with death. A carer should always check out the particular requirements, and respect the wishes of the dying person and the relatives.

 Key points

- Everyone has physical and psychological needs, and we develop drives which motivate us to fulfil those needs.
- A balanced diet is one that contains the complete range of foods in the correct proportions to meet the body's requirements.
- Different groups of people have different beliefs about the correct things to eat. These may be based on religion or philosophy.
- Infections are caused by pathogenic micro-organisms called bacteria and viruses.
- There are many ways to prevent infection including a healthy body, immunisations, good hygiene and effective public health measures.
- A strict method of hygiene, called barrier nursing, can be used to prevent the spread of some serious infections such as gastro-enteritis.
- Cleanliness is important to protect the skin and hair against damage or infection, but individual wishes must be respected.
- Frequent changing of position is one of the best safeguards in the prevention of pressure sores, together with a clean, dry skin.
- Continence can be encouraged through providing privacy, convenient toilet facilities, good communications, correct diet and fluids, exercise and care with certain drugs.
- Aids can be used for people who are incontinent in order to protect their skin and preserve their dignity. These include sheaths for men, pads and pants, and indwelling catheters.
- Independence can be encouraged through the use of a variety of aids and gadgets that help with mobility and daily living tasks.
- There are many safety features that can be incorporated into homes and the environment to protect people from injuries through accidents.
- Physical, psychological and social activities are important aspects of recreation, and help to keep both body and mind fit and healthy.
- Approaching and after death, people can go through four stages of bereavement: anticipation, shock, anger and acceptance.
- There are many customs associated with death, and the carer should check on the wishes of the individual and the relatives before death occurs.
- All individuals have their own beliefs and the carer should always respect these, and adjust their communications, behaviour and treatments to fit in with these beliefs and customs.

Appendix

A typical social services department structure

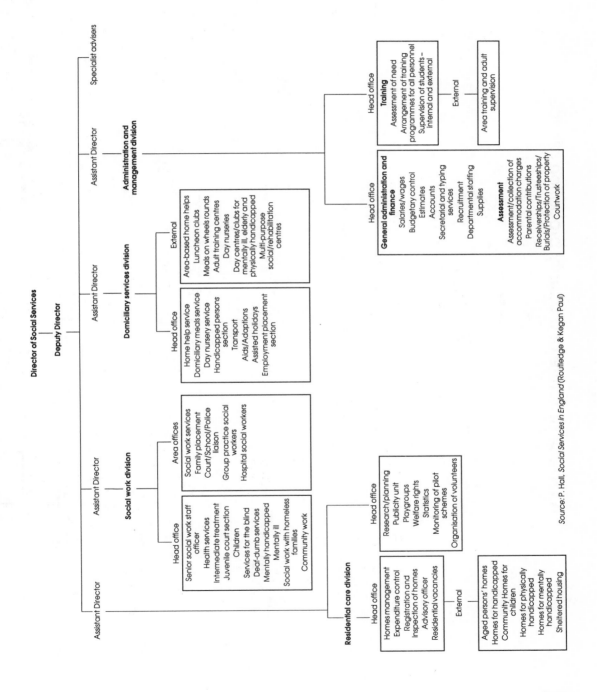

Director of Social Services

Deputy Director

Assistant Director | Assistant Director | Assistant Director | Assistant Director | Specialist advisers

Social work division

Area offices
Social work services
Family placement
Court/School/Police liaison
Group practice social workers
Hospital social workers

Head office
Senior social work staff officer
Health services
Intermediate treatment
Juvenile court section
Children
Services for the blind
Deaf-dumb services
Mentally ill
Mentally handicapped
Social work with homeless families
Community work

Residential care division

Head office
Research/planning
Publicity unit
Playgroups
Welfare rights
Statistics
Monitoring of pilot schemes
Organisation of volunteers

Head office
Homes management
Expenditure control
Registration and inspection of homes
Advisory officer
Residential vacancies

External
Aged persons' homes
Homes for handicapped
Community Homes for children
Homes for physically handicapped
Homes for mentally handicapped
Sheltered housing

Domiciliary services division

Head office
Home help service
Domiciliary meals service
Day nursery service
Handicapped persons section
Transport
Aids/Adaptions
Assisted holidays
Employment placement section

External
Area-based home helps
Luncheon clubs
Meals on wheels rounds
Adult training centres
Day nurseries
Day centres/clubs for mentally ill, elderly and physically handicapped
Multi-purpose social/rehabilitation centres

Administration and management division

Head office

General administration and finance
Salaries/wages
Budgetary control
Estimates
Accounts
Secretarial and typing services
Recruitment
Departmental staffing
Supplies

Assessment
Assessment/collection of accommodation charges
Parental contributions
Receiverships/Trusteeships/Burials/Protection of property
Courtwork

Head office

Training
Assessment of need
Arrangement of training programmes for all personnel
Supervision of students – internal and external

External
Area training and adult supervision

Source: P. Hall, Social Services in England (Routledge & Kegan Paul)

193

A typical structure of a county probation service

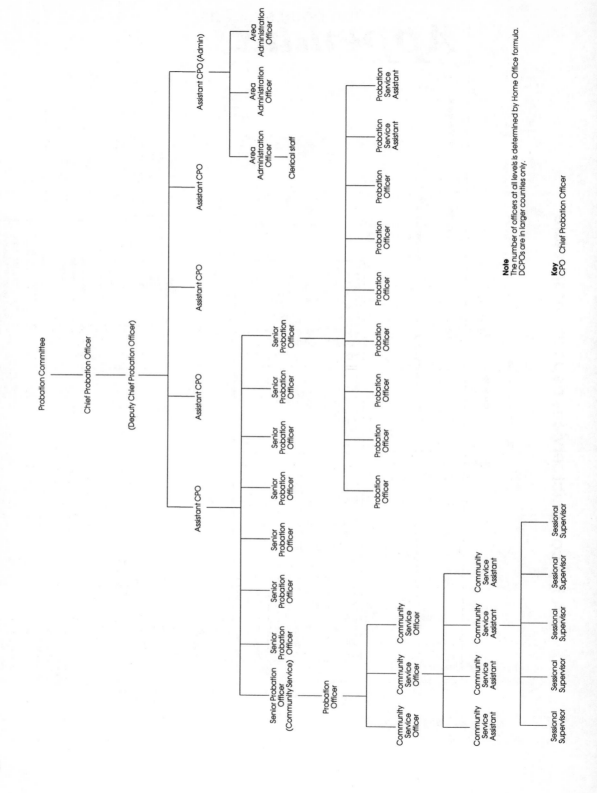

Note
The number of officers at all levels is determined by Home Office formula. DCPOs are in larger counties only.

Key
CPO   Chief Probation Officer

The court structure

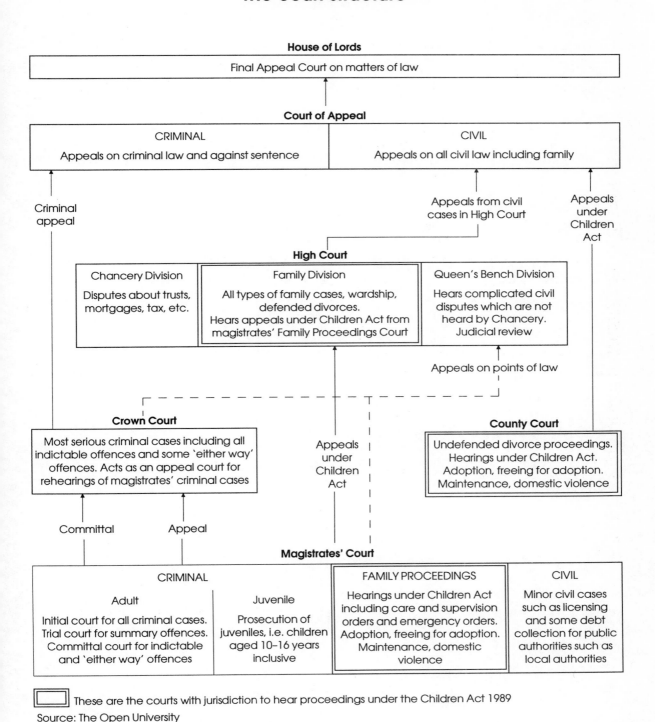

House of Lords

Final Appeal Court on matters of law

Court of Appeal

CRIMINAL	CIVIL
Appeals on criminal law and against sentence	Appeals on all civil law including family

Criminal appeal

Appeals from civil cases in High Court

Appeals under Children Act

High Court

Chancery Division	Family Division	Queen's Bench Division
Disputes about trusts, mortgages, tax, etc.	All types of family cases, wardship, defended divorces. Hears appeals under Children Act from magistrates' Family Proceedings Court	Hears complicated civil disputes which are not heard by Chancery. Judicial review

Appeals on points of law

Crown Court

Most serious criminal cases including all indictable offences and some 'either way' offences. Acts as an appeal court for rehearings of magistrates' criminal cases

Appeals under Children Act

County Court

Undefended divorce proceedings. Hearings under Children Act. Adoption, freeing for adoption. Maintenance, domestic violence

Committal   Appeal

Magistrates' Court

CRIMINAL		FAMILY PROCEEDINGS	CIVIL
Adult	Juvenile	Hearings under Children Act including care and supervision orders and emergency orders. Adoption, freeing for adoption. Maintenance, domestic violence	Minor civil cases such as licensing and some debt collection for public authorities such as local authorities
Initial court for all criminal cases. Trial court for summary offences. Committal court for indictable and 'either way' offences	Prosecution of juveniles, i.e. children aged 10–16 years inclusive		

These are the courts with jurisdiction to hear proceedings under the Children Act 1989

Source: The Open University

Glossary

Acquired disabilities Those that occur after birth, either through accidental injury or illness.

Adolescence The period of development between being a child and being grown up. Can be a time of turbulence and rebellion.

Agenda A list of business items to be discussed at a meeting.

Alzheimer's disease A progressive, degenerative disorder in which the nerve cells in the brain degenerate and the brain shrinks. It is the commonest cause of dementia.

Anaemia Blood disorders, in which the levels of the oxygen-carrying pigment, haemoglobin, are below normal.

Angina A painful condition caused by a restriction or narrowing of the arteries leading to the heart muscle. Pain is felt in the chest and left arm.

Antibiotics Drugs given to destroy pathogenic (disease-causing) organisms, such as bacteria, in the body.

Anti-discriminatory practice Promoting good care practice without making any differences between service users on grounds of gender, age, sex, race, religion and so on.

Anxiety An emotional state ranging from mild unease to intense fear. It becomes a problem when it inhibits or disrupts normal activities.

Arthritis A condition of the joints where the surfaces of the bones become worn causing pain and inflammation.

Asthma Attacks of breathlessness accompanied by wheezing, often caused by an allergy, but made worse by stress or anxiety.

Bacteria A group of single-celled micro-organisms, some of which may cause disease. *See* **Pathogens**.

Balanced diet A diet containing all the essential foods in the correct proportions for the individual.

Bereavement Feeling of desolation following death of someone close, or perhaps following the loss of limb.

Beri-beri A disease affecting the nervous system that occurs through a deficiency of Vitamin B.

Cancer Any of a group of diseases caused through the unrestrained growth of a particular group of cells, which may form growths or tumours. May cause leukaemia if occurring in the cells that form the blood cells.

Care plan A combination of services designed to meet the assessed needs of a person requiring care in the community.

Carer Any person providing care. Informal carers may be members of the family or a friend; professional carers are employed by one of the service providers.

Carriers People who carry pathogenic organisms, passing them on to others, but not necessarily showing signs of the disease themselves.

Case conference A meeting involving a range of professional people (social worker, doctor, teacher, foster-parent and so on) who meet together to discuss the needs of a client for the future.

Census An information-gathering exercise carried out for the government to gain facts about the total population.

Channel of communication The means of communication through which messages flow from source to destination. Most examples of the communication process involve multiple (or many) channels.

Chemotherapy The treatment of conditions by chemical substances.

Chiropody Diagnosis, treatment and prevention of diseases and malfunctions of the foot.

Confidentiality Protecting a client's/patient's rights to secrecy and not divulging any information which is given in confidence by that person.

Congenital disabilities Those that people are born with.

Consultant A physician or surgeon holding the highest appointment in a particular branch of surgery or medicine in a hospital.

Continence The ability to control the passing of urine and faeces, in other words controlling the bladder and bowel functions.

Contraception The prevention of conception (fertilisation of an ovum) or pregnancy, by barrier, hormonal or sterilisation methods.

Cultural deprivation A person who is unaware of their cultural origins or who is denied the right to practise their cultural beliefs, values or behaviours.

Culture A collection of beliefs, values and behaviours which are distinctive to a large group of people and are expressed through language, dress, religion, music and art forms. Culture is often identified in terms of a nation.

Cystitis Inflammation of the bladder, causing pain and frequency in passing urine.

Degenerative disorders Conditions in which there is a progressive impairment of the functioning of a part of the body. It may be due to age, infection, inflammation, chemical or physical damage.

Dementia A general decline in all mental abilities.

Depression Feelings of sadness, hopelessness and a general loss of interest in life. This state occurs normally as a response to an event such as bereavement. If it occurs without any apparent cause, or it deepens and persists, it is classified as a psychiatric illness.

Dermatitis Inflammation of the skin, often due to an allergy.

Disability (World Health Organisation definition) Any restriction or lack (resulting from an impairment) of ability to perform an activity in the manner or within the range considered normal for a human being.

Dominant genes Those genes carrying characteristics which appear in the offspring.

Drives The forces that drive individuals to behaviours that enable their needs to be met.

Enema A procedure in which fluid is passed through a tube, inserted into the anus (rectum). Usually done to clear the intestine of faeces.

Extended family A sociological term referring to a social unit which consists of mother, father and children who either live with, or are in close proximity to, grandparents, aunts, uncles, cousins etc. Families often span three or more generations, often under one roof.

Feedback In communication terms feedback is the response to a previous message. It includes the idea that the sender adjusts their communication style or method in response to feedback. Feedback is continuous in a conversation. Feedback can be an intentional response in terms of a spoken reply or it can be unintentional in terms of some non-verbal behaviours.

Fibroid A benign or non-malignant tumour in the uterus.

Franglais Informal words included in the French language which are of English derivation, e.g. *le weekend, le camping*.

Genetic Things that are inherited from parents, through genes or the units of inheritance.

Genetic counselling An advisory service for people who think they may carry the risk of passing on an inherited or genetic disorder to any children they may have.

Guthrie test A blood test carried out routinely on young babies in order to detect phenylketonuria, an inherited disorder that can lead to brain damage unless treated. Normally the baby's heel is pricked and a few drops of blood are soaked into absorbent paper, which is then tested.

Haemoglobin The oxygen carrying pigment in the red blood corpuscles.

Half-way hostels Hostels provided by housing departments and associations to house homeless people before they are offered more permanent accommodation.

Handicap (World Health Organisation definition) A disadvantage for a given individual, resulting from an impairment or disability, that limits or prevents the fulfilment of a role, depending on age, sex, and social and cultural factors, for that individual.

Health visitor A nurse employed by a district health authority to visit people in their own homes, and give help and advice on health and welfare issues to particular social groupings including mothers with pre-school children and elderly people. They are qualified nurses and midwives and hold a health visitor's certificate.

Hospice A residential care setting (often in the private or voluntary sector), specialising in the care of people with terminal illnesses.

HRT Hormone replacement therapy, a relatively new drug therapy given to women at the time of the menopause in order to counteract some of the effects of hormone deficiency, such as osteoporosis.

Hysteria A general term used to describe a number of disorders including amnesia. Mass hysteria can occur as a group response to tensions or worries.

Immunisation The process of inducing immunity or protection against an infective disease such as tetanus.

Impairment (World Health Organisation definition) Any loss or abnormality of psychological, physiological or anatomical structure or function.

Income support A means-tested cash benefit which replaced supplementary benefit and is claimed by people whose cash resources fall below a certain level set each year by the government.

Incontinence Having no control over bladder and/or bowel function, therefore not being able to control the flow of urine or the passing of faeces.

Insight Understanding of hidden situations and/or characters.

Intuition Immediate understanding without reasoning.

Jargon A specialised language concerned with a particular subject, culture or profession.

Judiciary The judges of a state.

Key worker A named member of staff who has primary contact with a resident or service user and their family.

Labelling An analysis of social processes involved in the social attribution of positive, or more usually, negative characteristics to acts, individuals or groups within society.

Makaton A simple sign language used with hearing-impaired people and those with a learning disability who may find it difficult to communicate.

Manic depression Severe disturbance of mood, ranging from depression to mania or elation.

Metabolism The process of using food or nutrition to meet the body's needs.

Minutes A written record of the decisions reached at a meeting.

Mode of communication A 'language' for getting a message across to the sender, e.g. sign language, music or a painting. Both sender and receiver need to understand the 'language' which is being used.

Monogamous Being married to, or having a relationship with, one partner at a time.

Motives The reasons why individuals behave in a particular manner.

National insurance contributions Sums of money deducted at source, weekly or monthly, from people who are in employment, to finance the National Health Service and other social care benefits for sick, unemployed, elderly people and so on.

Needs Basic needs are all those things that individuals need to have met in order to survive, e.g. hunger.

Nephritis Inflammation in the kidney often caused by infection.

Neuritis Inflammation of a nerve or nerves.

Neuroses Mild forms of psychiatric disorders in which the individual remains in contact with reality.

Non-pathogenic Micro-organisms which are present but do not cause disease, in fact may have a beneficial effect.

Non-verbal communication A means of communication which includes body language, paralanguage and dress. *See **Paralanguage**.*

Nuclear family A sociological term referring to a family unit consisting of mother, father and at least one child.

Occupational therapist A qualified therapist who helps elderly, handicapped and mentally ill people, and people with learning disabilities by advising about aids for mobility and creative crafts etc., in order to help them recover or live more fulfilled lives.

Orchitis An inflammation of the testis.

Osteomalacia A weakening or softening of the bones of adults due to a deficiency in vitamin D. In children the condition is called rickets.

Osteoporosis Loss of protein from the bones, causing them to become brittle and easily fractured. It is a natural part of the ageing process, but early osteoporosis is more likely to occur in women after the menopause, due to the decrease in the hormone levels.

Paralanguage The non-verbal signs which accompany speech, for example a gasp, or an 'er' or 'um'. They can be clues to interpret the non-verbal communication.

Paraplegia Paralysis of both legs and sometimes part of the lower trunk, due to damage of the spinal cord.

Parkinson's disease A neurological disorder causing tremors, stiffness and weakness, resulting in slow movements and a shuffling, unbalanced walk. It is a degenerative disease affecting about 1 in 200 people in the UK.

Pathogens Micro-organisms that cause disease.

Peer group People from the same grouping. May be based on many characteristics, including class, interest, occupations, age.

Pellagra A nutritional disorder caused by deficiency of one of the vitamin B complex, niacin, often occurring in countries where the staple diet is maize.

Pernicious anaemia A type of anaemia caused by deficiency in vitamin B_{12}.

Phobia A persistent, irrational fear.

Physical Associated with the body.

Physiotherapy Treating of disorders or injuries through physical methods such as exercise, massage, heat treatment or hydrotherapy.

Pneumonia An infection of the lung causing inflammation. It is a common late complication of many illnesses, causing about 27,000 deaths a year in the UK.

Poverty line An imaginary line representing a minimum income level, below which people who do not have very much live. People below the poverty line are sometimes referred to as those who are dependent on income support and who have to live at a standard below this imaginary line.

Practice nurse A registered general nurse who works within a general practice with a group of general practitioners.

Primary socialisation Process by which a child learns about the society/culture they are growing up in from their family including brothers and sisters etc.

Private A caring/medical service which is set up in order to make a profit.

Prostate gland A solid, chestnut-shaped organ surrounding the first part of the urethra in the male, situated under the bladder and in front of the rectum. In older men it may become enlarged and interface with the passing of urine.

Psychological Associated with the functioning of the abstract processes of the brain, such as intelligence.

Psychoses Severe psychiatric disorders in which the individual loses contact with reality.

Puberty Becoming functionally capable of reproduction through natural development of reproductive organs.

Radiotherapy The treatment of conditions by the use of radioactivity, such as X-rays.

Ramadan The ninth month of the Muslim year, during which rigid fasting is observed during all daylight hours.

Recessive gene One that carries characteristics which will only appear in the offspring if matched with another recessive gene. If paired with a dominant gene the trait is concealed, and the characteristics of the dominant gene are the ones that appear.

Renal dialysis A method of treatment for people with kidney failure. The blood is passed through a 'kidney machine' which extracts the waste products before the blood is returned to the individual.

Respite care A service provided usually for informal carers. The person they care for may be offered short-term residential care or professional carers may come into the home to provide a break for the relatives or friends of the service user.

Schizophrenia A general term for a group of psychotic illnesses in which the individual has disturbances of thinking, emotional reaction and behaviour. Thoughts, behaviour and feelings do not relate to each other, hence the 'split personality'.

Scurvy Caused by a deficiency in vitamin C, this condition is characterised by bruising, haemorrhaging and painful joints.

Secondary socialisation Process by which a child learns about the society/culture they are growing up in from sub-cultures external to the family, e.g. nursery, school, peers etc.

Self-concept The way people see themselves.

Self-esteem The way in which we think of ourselves which in turn affects our self-image.

Self-image A view of ourselves as we see ourselves and not as others see us.

Septicaemia Commonly known as blood poisoning, when there is a rapid multiplication of bacteria and their toxins in the blood.

Service user Someone who receives or uses social or health care services. Also referred to as a client or patient.

Sexually transmitted diseases Diseases that are transmitted or passed from one human being to another through sexual activity.

Shingles An infection of the nerves that supply certain areas of the skin, causing a very painful rash of small, crusting blisters. It is caused by the same virus as chicken-pox.

Single-parent family A family in which any children are being brought up by one parent, either male or female.

Social class The hierarchical distinctions which exist between individuals or groups with a society.

Socialisation Process in which culture of society is transmitted to children.

Sociology The systematic study of the functioning organisations and different types of human society.

Special needs The needs that people with disabilities have.

Special school A school which provides education for children with a disability or learning difficulties. It may be a day school or a school where some children board during the week and go home to families at the weekend.

Statutory A service or provision which has to be made by statute law.

Step-parent families A family in which either mother or father has remarried and brought to the new family unit child(ren) from a previous marriage.

Stereotype A set of inaccurate, simple generalisations about a group of individuals which enables others to categorise members of this group and treat them according to their expectations. Race, social class and gender stereotypes are commonly held, and lead to the perception and treatment of others according the unjustified beliefs.

Stroke A condition where part of the brain has a restricted blood supply due to a clot or haemorrhage in one of the brain's blood vessels. Technically known as a cerebro-vascular accident or CVA.

Sub-culture Any system of beliefs, values or norms which is shared and actively participated in by a minority of people within a culture.

Substance abuse The use of substances, such as drugs or glue, that cause one of many effects, including a sense of well-being or hallucinations.

Supervision order An order made by the courts in respect of a young person under the Children Act 1989. The young person remains in their own home but is the subject of supervision by a social worker. Either a condition or intermediate treatment can be attached to a supervision order.

Suppository A solid cone or bullet-shaped object which may contain a drug. It is inserted into the rectum, where it melts. It may be used to soften